Problem Solvi

Problem Solving in
Acute Oncology

Edited by

Ernie Marshall, MD, MRCP(UK), MBChB
Macmillian Consultant in Medical Oncology, Clatterbridge Cancer Centre,
Merseyside, UK

Alison Young, MD, MRCP(UK), MBChB
Consultant Medical Oncologist, St James's Institute of Oncology, St James's
University Hospital, Leeds, UK

Peter I. Clark, MA MD FRCP
Professor of Medical Oncology, Clatterbridge Cancer Centre Merseyside, UK;
Chair of NHS England Chemotherapy Clinical Reference Group

Peter Selby, CBE, DSc, MD, FRCP FRCR FMedSci
Professor of Cancer Medicine, St James's Institute of Oncology and University of
Leeds, Leeds, UK; President of the Association of Cancer Physicians

Published in association with the Association of Cancer Physicians

CLINICAL PUBLISHING
OXFORD

CLINICAL PUBLISHING
an imprint of Atlas Medical Publishing Ltd
110 Innovation House, Parkway Court
Oxford Business Park South, Oxford OX4 0JY

Tel: +44 1865 811116
Fax: +44 1865 251550

E mail: info@clinicalpublishing.co.uk
Web: www.clinicalpublishing.co.uk

Distributed in USA and Canada by:
Clinical Publishing
30 Amberwood Parkway
Ashland OH 44805 USA
tel: 800-247-6553 (toll free within US and Canada)
fax: 419-281-6883
email: order@bookmasters.com

Distributed in UK and Rest of World by:
Marston Book Services Ltd
PO Box 269
Abingdon
Oxon OX14 4YN UK
tel: +44 1235 465500
fax: +44 1235 465555
email: trade.orders@marston.co.uk

© Atlas Medical Publishing Ltd 2014

First published 2014

A catalogue record for this book is available from the British Library.

ISBN 13   978 1 84692 108 7
ISBN e-book 978 1 84692 649 5

Series design by Pete Russell Typographic Design, Faringdon, Oxon., UK
Typeset by Ian Winter Design, Ramsden, Oxon., UK
Printed by Latimer Trend and Company Ltd, Plymouth, UK

Contents

SECTION ONE   Perspectives in the Development of Acute Oncology

SECTION TWO   Complications of Systemic Therapy

SECTION THREE Complications of Radiotherapy

SECTION FOUR Complications of Cancer

SECTION FIVE Acute Palliative Care and Pain Control

SECTION SIX Patients in Clinical Trials

Contributors

Dr Shaker Abdallah, Consultant Medical Oncologist, Clatterbridge Cancer Centre, Merseyside

Dr Mehran Afshar , Specialist Registrar in Medical Oncology, St James's Institute of Oncology, Leeds

Dr Eliyaz Ahmed, Consultant Medical Oncologist, Clatterbridge Cancer Centre, Merseyside

Dr Alan Anthoney, Consultant Medical Oncologist, St James's Institute of Oncology, Leeds

Dr Mary Anthonypillai, Specialist Registrar in Clinical Oncology, Clatterbridge Cancer Centre, Merseyside

Mrs Maxine Armitage, Clinical Nurse Specialist in Haematology/Oncology, Airedale General Hospital, Keighley

Mrs Debbie Beirne, Nurse Consultant, St James's Institute of Oncology, Leeds

Professor Michael Bennett, Professor of Palliative Medicine, Leeds Institute of Health Sciences, Leeds

Professor Julia Newton Bishop, Professor of Dermatology, University of Leeds, Leeds

Mr Andrew Brodbelt, Consultant Neurosurgeon, Walton Centre, Liverpool, Merseyside

Dr Janet Brown, Consultant Medical Oncologist, St James's Institute of Oncology, Leeds

Dr Judith Carser, Consultant Medical Oncologist, Clatterbridge Cancer Centre, Merseyside

Dr Madhuchanda Chatterjee, Specialist Registrar in Clinical Oncology, Clatterbridge Cancer Centre, Merseyside

Dr Fiona Collinson, Consultant Medical Oncologist, St James's Institute of Oncology, Leeds

Professor Gordon Cook, Professor of Haematology, St James's Institute of Oncology, Leeds

Dr Michael Crawford, Consultant Medical Oncologist, Airedale General Hospital, Keighley

Dr Luis Daverede, Specialist Registrar in Medical Oncology, St James's Institute of Oncology, Leeds

Mr Sean Duffy, NCD for Cancer, NHS England

Mrs Patricia Dyminski, Lead Clinical Nurse Specialist in Haematology/Oncology, Airedale General Hospital, Keighley

Dr Amy Ford, Specialist Registrar in Medical Oncology, Clatterbridge Cancer Centre, Merseyside

Dr Helen Ford, Consultant Neurologist, Leeds Teaching Hospitals NHS Trust, Leeds

Dr Maged Gharib, Consultant Haematologist, St Helens & Knowsley Hospital, Merseyside

Dr Stephen Gilbey, Consultant Endocrinologist, Leeds Teaching Hospitals NHS Trust, Leeds

Dr John Green, Consultant Medical Oncologist, Clatterbridge Cancer Centre, Merseyside

Dr Richard Griffiths, Consultant Medical Oncologist, Clatterbridge Cancer Centre, Merseyside

Dr Allison Hall, Consultant Clinical Oncologist, Clatterbridge Cancer Centre, Merseyside

Dr Anoop Haridass, Specialist Registrar in Clinical Oncology, Clatterbridge Cancer Centre, Merseyside

Dr Ahmed Hashmim, Specialist Registrar in Clinical Oncology, Clatterbridge Cancer Centre, Merseyside

Dr Greg Heath, Specialist Registrar in Medical Ophthalmology, Yorkshire Deanery

Dr Adam Hurlow, Consultant in Palliative Medicine, Leeds Teaching Hospitals NHS Trust, Leeds

Dr Helen Innes, Consultant Medical Oncologist, Clatterbridge Cancer Centre, Merseyside

Dr Pooja Jain, Consultant Clinical Oncologist, Clatterbridge Cancer Centre, Merseyside

Dr Adel Jebar, Specialist Registrar in Medical Oncology, St James's Institute of Oncology, Leeds

Dr Rebecca Jones, Consultant Hepatologist, Leeds Teaching Hospitals NHS Trust, Leeds

Mr Neil Kapoor, Consultant Gastroenterologist, Aintree University Hospital, Merseyside

Dr Monika Krzyzanowska, Associate Professor of Medicine, Princess Margaret Cancer Centre, Toronto, Canada

Dr Martin Ledson, Consultant Respiratory Physician, Liverpool Heart and Chest Hospital, Merseyside

Dr Daniel Lee, Specialist Registrar in Medical Oncology, St James's Institute of Oncology, Leeds

Dr Pauline Leonard, Consultant Medical Oncologist, Whittington Health, London

Dr Andrew Lewington, Consultant Renal Physician, Leeds Teaching Hospitals NHS Trust, Leeds

Dr Ernie Marshall, Macmillian Consultant in Medical Oncology, Clatterbridge Cancer Centre, Merseyside

Dr Jennifer Malin, Medical Director, Oncology, WellPoint, Inc, Thousand Oaks, CA, USA

Dr Sid McNulty, Consultant Endocrinologist, St Helen's & Knowsley Hospital, Merseyside

Dr Nabile Mohsin, Consultant Radiologist, St Helen's & Knowsley Hospital, Merseyside

Dr Anna Mullard, Specialist Registrar in Medical Oncology, Clatterbridge Cancer Centre, Merseyside

Dr Stuart Murdoch, Consultant Anaesthetist, Leeds Teaching Hospitals NHS Trust, Leeds

Dr Jay Naik, Consultant Medical Oncologist, Mid Yorkshire Hospitals NHS Trust, Wakefield

Dr Karen Neoh, Academic Clinical Fellow in Palliative Medicine, Leeds Institute of Health Sciences, Leeds

Dr Helen Neville-Webbe, Consultant Medical Oncologist, Clatterbridge Cancer Centre, Merseyside

Ms Kathryn Oddy, Matron for Oncology, St James's Institute of Oncology, Leeds

Dr Richard Osborne, Consultant Medical Oncologist, Dorset Cancer Centre, Poole

Dr Lisa Owen, Specialist Registrar in Clinical Oncology, St James's Institute of Oncology, Leeds

Dr Nick Palmer, Consultant Cardiologist, Liverpool Heart and Chest Hospital, Merseyside

Dr Christopher Parrish, Specialist Registrar in Haematology, Leeds Teaching Hospitals NHS Trust, Leeds

Dr Paul Plant, Consultant Chest Physician, Leeds Teaching Hospitals NHS Trust, Leeds

Dr Chris Plummer, Consultant Cardiologist, Freeman Hospital, Newcastle upon Tyne

Dr Anthony Pope, Consultant Clinical Oncologist, Clatterbridge Cancer Centre, Merseyside

Dr Pankaj Punia, Specialist Registrar in Medical Oncology, St James's Institute of Oncology, Leeds

Dr Christy Ralph, Consultant Medical Oncologist, St James's Institute of Oncology, Leeds

Dr Satiavani Ramasamy, Specialist Registrar in Clinical Oncology, St James's Institute of Oncology, Leeds

Dr Emma Rathbone, Specialist Registrar in Medical Oncology, St James's Institute of Oncology, Leeds

Dr Komal Ray, Specialist Registrar in Anaesthetics, Leeds Teaching Hospitals NHS Trust, Leeds

Mrs Jeanette Ribton, Acute Oncology Lead Nurse, St Helen's & Knowsley Hospital, Merseyside

Professor Sir Michael Richards, Chief Inspector of Hospitals, Care Quality Commission

Professor Bridget Robinson, Professor in Cancer Medicine, Christchurch Hospital, Christchurch, New Zealand

Dr Peter Robson, Consultant Clinical Oncologist, Clatterbridge Cancer Centre, Merseyside

Mr Mike Scott, Consultant Colorectal Surgeon, St Helen's & Knowsley Hospital, Merseyside

Dr Jenny Seligmann, Specialist Registrar in Medical Oncology, St James's Institute of Oncology, Leeds

Professor Susan Short, Professor of Clinical Oncology and Neuro-Oncology, St James's Institute of Oncology, Leeds

Dr Cath Siller, Consultant Medical Oncologist, Mid Yorkshire Hospitals NHS Trust, Wakefield

Dr Dan Stark, Consultant Medical Oncologist, St James's Institute of Oncology, Leeds

Dr Dan Swinson, Consultant Medical Oncologist, St James's Institute of Oncology, Leeds

Dr Isabel Syndikus, Consultant Clinical Oncologist, Clatterbridge Cancer Centre, Merseyside

Dr Chan Ton, Consultant Medical Oncologist, Clatterbridge Cancer Centre, Merseyside

Professor Chris Twelves, Professor of Clinical Cancer Pharmacology and Oncology, St James's Institute of Oncology, Leeds

Dr Gordon Urquhart, Specialist Registrar in Medical Oncology, St James's Institute of Oncology, Leeds

Dr Jennifer Walsh, Consultant in Endocrinology and Metabolic Bone Medicine, Sheffield Teaching Hospitals, Sheffield

Dr Jonathan Wide, Consultant Radiologist, St Helen's & Knowsley Hospital, Merseyside

Mr Martin Wilby, Consultant Neurosurgeon, The Walton Centre, Liverpool, Merseyside

Dr Charlie Wilkinson, Consultant in Acute and Elderly Medicine, Leeds Teaching Hospitals NHS Trust, Leeds

Dr Lucy Wyld, Specialist Registrar in Medical Oncology, St James's Institute of Oncology, Leeds

Dr Alison Young, Consultant Medical Oncologist, St James's Institute of Oncology, Leeds

Foreword

The Importance of Acute Oncology to Cancer Patients

We have made considerable progress to improve the services provided in the NHS for cancer patients. Multidisciplinary specialized care has been developed throughout the NHS, and cancer services have been reconfigured to ensure that patients move to the appropriate place so that their care can be provided by teams with the right specialized expertise. Facilities have been improved and there have been substantial increases in workforce and training. These developments have not completed the task. We have much to do to maintain and continue to improve the excellence of care and to ensure that patients can quickly and appropriately gain access to that care. Although cancer outcomes in the UK are getting better, there is room for further improvement.

Emergency presentation as the route to diagnosis for cancer is common. In England, 24% of all cancers present in this way and the proportion is greater in patients over 70 years of age. For all cancers emergency presentation is associated with a poorer outcome and patients are less likely to survive the next year following presentation.

The development of acute oncology will improve the care of cancer patients, the management of acute complications of cancer, and of its treatment, and our approaches to diagnosing patients who present with cancer and have no obvious primary site. This will address the needs of patients who present acutely to the healthcare system with findings that suggest the possibility of a malignancy, ensure that patients who develop acute complications of their cancer or their treatment are seen, evaluated and managed promptly by clinicians with the right skills and facilities, and provide a supportive acute cancer care service for patients throughout their journey. Key appointments in acute oncology, many at consultant and nurse practitioner level, are being made across the NHS.

There remains a need to ensure that practitioners are fully informed and kept up to date with the appropriate clinical care to be provided in the setting of acute oncology. It is also necessary to ensure a continuing developmental dialogue on the best way to deliver acute oncology services in a hard-pressed healthcare service. For these reasons, this text on acute oncology is particularly helpful and timely. It will serve as a valuable resource for those who have to continue to develop an excellent acute oncology service, as well as providing a source of training and updates for clinicians working in this challenging clinical area. The Association of Cancer Physicians is to be congratulated on bringing about this valuable additional resource, which is the first of its kind, and we can look forward to further contributions in future.

Michael Richards, Sean Duffy

Preface

Michael Richards and Sean Duffy, who lead the development of cancer care in the UK, have drawn attention to the importance of acute oncology in providing high-quality cancer care for our patients. We have prepared this book in the format of the *Problem Solving* series in order to present the issues surrounding the development of acute oncology services, both in the UK and internationally, in a patient-centred format. We have illustrated most of the problems that will present to an oncologist who is part of the acute oncology services. These cover the perspective of service development, but also many aspects of acute general medical and acute oncological care that will arise, this includes the care of patients with cancer of unknown primary site, the major complications of systemic therapy (especially febrile neutropenia), the complications of radiotherapy, the major acute complications of cancer itself and some considerations of patients in clinical trials presenting acutely. Palliative care and pain control can be critically important challenges to oncology services, and key aspects of these are set out in the context of patient related-problems.

Our purpose is to provide a highly patient-centred, readable text, that will support acute oncologists both in training and in practice. We hope that it will provide a valuable resource for all acute oncology services to those who are charged with developing acute oncology services in the future across the world, and be helpful for the individual oncologist, whether in training or established as consultants and staff physicians. Acute oncology has been developing rapidly, bringing improvements in services and benefits to patients. We hope this book will help this process and add to its momentum.

Ernie Marshall, Alison Young, Peter Clark and Peter Selby

Acknowledgements

The editors warmly acknowledge the support they have received in preparing this book. Nicole Goldman coordinated and oversaw the book's preparation and organization.

The editors, authors and the publisher are most grateful to Dr Johnathan Joffe, the Chairman of the ACP, and the ACP Executive for their support and advice during the development of this book.

Abbreviations

ACE	angiotensin-converting enzyme	DM	diabetes mellitus
ADLs	activities of daily living	DPP-4	dipeptidyl peptidase 4
AE	adverse event	DPYD	dihydropyrimidine dehydrogenase
AKI	acute kidney injury	DVT	deep vein thrombosis
ALF	acute liver failure	EC	epirubicin and cyclophosphamide
ALP	alkaline phosphatase	ECG	electrocardiogram
ALT	alanine transaminase	ECOG	Eastern Cooperative Oncology
AOS	acute oncology service(s)		Group
AOT	acute oncology team	ED	emergency department
AR	adverse reaction	EDTA	ethylenediaminetetraacetic acid
ASCO	American Society of Clinical	EGFR	epidermal growth factor receptor
	Oncology	FBC	full blood count
AST	aspartate transaminase	FEC	fluorouracil, epirubicin and
bpm	beats per minute		cyclophosphamide
BCNU	bis-chloroethylnitrosourea	5-FU	fluorouracil
	(carmustine)	FNA	fine-needle aspiration
CA125	cancer antigen 125	GCP	good clinical practice
	(MUC16, mucin 16)	G-CSF	granulocyte colony-stimulating
CCC	Clatterbridge Cancer Centre		factor
CEA	carcinoembryonic antigen	GEBP	gene expression-based profiling
CFS	cerebrospinal fluid	GFR	glomerular filtration rate
CHF	congestive heart failure	GI	gastrointestinal
CID	chemotherapy-induced diarrhoea	GIST	gastrointestinal stromal tumour
CKD	chronic kidney disease	GLP-1	glucagon-like peptide-1
CNS	central nervous system	GP	general practitioner
CONcePT	Comparison of Oxaliplatin vs	Hb	haemoglobin concentration
	Conventional Methods with	HbA1c	glycosylated haemoglobin
	Calcium/Magnesium in First-Line	HBcAg	core antigen of hepatitis B virus
	Metastatic Colorectal Cancer	HBeAg	core antigen of hepatitis B virus,
	(NCT00129870)		extracellular form
COPD	chronic obstructive pulmonary	HBsAg	surface antigen of hepatitis B virus
	disease	HBV	hepatitis B virus
COSA	Clinical Oncology Society of	HER2	human epidermal growth factor
	Australia		receptor 2
CPAP	continuous positive airway	HFS	hand-foot syndrome
	pressure	HSCT	haematopoietic stem cell
Cr	creatinine		transplantation
CRF	case record form	IB	Investigator Brochure
CT	computed tomography	IDSA	Infectious Diseases Society of
CTCAE	Common Terminology Criteria for		America
	Adverse Events	IgE	immunoglobulin E
CUP	cancer of unknown primary	IMRT	intensity-modulated radiation
CVP	central venous pressure		therapy
DGH	district general hospital	INR	international normalized ratio

IV	intravenous	PPI	proton pump inhibitor
IVC	inferior vena cava	PQRI	Physician Quality Reporting
LEVF	left ventricular ejection fraction		Initiative
LMWH	low-molecular-weight heparin	PRES	posterior reversible
LN	lymph node		encephalopathy syndrome
MASCC	Multinational Association of	PSA	prostate-specific antigen
	Supportive Care in Cancer	PTHrP	parathyroid hormone-related
MCCN	Merseyside and Cheshire Cancer		protein
	Network	QOPI	Quality of Oncology Practice
MdG	modified de Gramont regimen		Initiative
MDT	multi disciplinary team	RCP	Royal College of Physicians
MOSAIC	Multicenter International Study of	RPA	recursive partitioning analysis
	Oxaliplatin/5FU-LV in the	RTK	receptor tyrosine kinase
	Adjuvant Treatment of Colon	RTOG	Radiation Therapy Oncology
	Cancer		Group
MRCC	metastatic renal cell carcinoma	RUL	right upper lobe
MRI	magnetic resonance imaging	SAAG	serum-ascites albumin gradient
MRSA	methicillin-resistant *Staphylococcus*	SACT	systemic anticancer therapy
	aureus	SAE	serious adverse event
MSCC	metastatic spinal cord compression	SAR	serious adverse reaction
MUO	malignancy of undefined primary	SCF	supraclavicular fossa
	origin	SCLC	small-cell lung cancer
NCAG	National Cancer Action Group	SIADH	syndrome of inappropriate
NCCTG	North Central Cancer Treatment		antidiuretic hormone
	Group	SJIO	St James's Institute of Oncology
NCEPOD	National Confidential Enquiry into	Sp_{O_2}	arterial oxygen saturation
	Patient Outcome and Death		measured by pulse oximetry
NCIN	National Cancer Intelligence	SpR	specialist registrar
	Network	SRS	stereotactic radiosurgery
NCQA	National Committee for Quality	SSG	site-specific group
	Assurance	SUSAR	suspected unexpected serious
NEWS	national early warning score		adverse reaction
NHS	National Health Service	SVCO	superior vena cava obstruction
NICE	National Institute for Health and	T4	levothyroxine
	Care Excellence	TKI	tyrosine kinase inhibitor
NNH	number needed to harm	TLS	tumour lysis syndrome
NNT	number needed to treat	U&Es	blood test for urea and electrolytes
NS	neutropenic sepsis		(sodium and potassium)
NYHA	New York Heart Association	UGT	uridine diphosphate-
OPD	outpatient department		glucuronosyltransferase
PCD	paraneoplastic cerebellar	UK	United Kingdom
	degeneration	Ur	supraclavicular fossa
PCN	percutaneous nephrostomy	US	United States (of America)
PDGF	platelet-derived growth factor	VATS	video-assisted thoracic surgery
PDGFR	PDGF receptor	VEGF	vascular endothelial growth factor
PE	pulmonary embolus	VEGFR	VEGF receptor
PET	positron emission tomography	VRE	vancomycin-resistant *Enterococcus*
PICC	peripherally inserted central	VTE	venous thromboembolism
	catheter	WBC	white blood cell count
PIS	patient information sheet	WBRT	whole-brain radiotherapy
P_{O_2}	oxygen tension (partial pressure)	WHO	World Health Organization

Perspectives in the Development of Acute Oncology

PROBLEM

01 The Development of Acute Oncology: Solutions and Options

Ernie Marshall, Pauline Leonard, Alison Young

Case Histories

Patient 1: A 74-year-old man presents to primary care with a three-month history of progressive lumbar spine pain despite analgesia and physiotherapy. The patient has localizing tenderness but no neurological deficit and this leads the GP to request an MRI spine. The MRI report is faxed urgently to primary care stating that there are findings consistent with multiple metastases present throughout the spine.

Patient 2: A 54-year-old woman with Grade 3, T2 N1 breast cancer is undergoing adjuvant FEC chemotherapy and develops nausea and dizziness. The patient is hypotensive with a temperature of 39°C and the GP requests an urgent ambulance to direct the patient to the nearest emergency department for review.

Patient 3: A 65-year-old woman, previously fit and well, presents to her local A&E department with acute abdominal pain, weight loss, anorexia, and increasing tiredness and lethargy. She is admitted acutely to the medical assessment unit and is found on CT scan to have liver metastases.

How do acute oncology models differ within and across cancer networks?

How would differing acute oncology models support the management of the above emergency presentations?

Background

Cancer is a major health issue. In the UK there are 325 000 new cases of cancer diagnosed annually. There are 157 000 deaths, contributing 28% of all deaths every year. With a wealth of possible curative and life-prolonging treatments it is estimated there are 1.7 million cancer survivors.[1]

The National Audit Office Hospital Episode Statistics estimate that the number of patients receiving systemic anticancer chemotherapy (SACT) has been increasing year on year since 2001/02, accounting for £1 billion expenditure annually.

The National Confidential Enquiry into Patient Outcome and Death (NCEPOD),[2] published in 2008, provided uncomfortable reading regarding the quality and safety of care for patients who died within 30 days of receiving SACT. The enquiry was set up especially to understand precisely the care pathways for this group of sick cancer patients. In only 35% of patients was the care deemed to be acceptable. In the 49% of patients where care was less than optimal, factors relating to both the organization of emergency care and the specific care delivered by each institution were identified. The National Chemotherapy Advisory Group (NCAG)[3] was formed to address how care should be delivered, not only to improve the outcome of the sick cancer patient, but to also address key issues in the organization of care to improve the patient experience.

The development of an Acute Oncology Service (AOS) in every trust with an emergency department was a key recommendation of the NCEPOD report. It described an AOS as one that brings together the expertise from oncology disciplines, emergency medicine, general medicine and general surgery to ensure the rapid identification and prompt management of all patients who present with severe complications following chemotherapy or as a consequence of their cancer. Uniquely, it also described the management of patients who present as emergencies with previously undiagnosed cancer as a key responsibility of an AOS. These groups of patients who present to the emergency department with a constellation of symptoms and are subsequently found to have cancer represent 22% of all new cancers diagnosed each year in England, with lung, pancreas and brain malignant tumours forming the largest group. Data collected by the National Cancer Intelligence Network (NCIN) have shown that, apart from acute leukaemia, the survival for this group of patients is far worse than for those who are referred by their general practitioner (GP) directly to elective non-emergency services. This is because such patients are usually of poor performance status, often elderly, and with multiple comorbidities. Their median survival is short as they are frequently too unwell to benefit from SACT or other potentially life-prolonging interventions. It was clear this group of patients needed properly coordinated pathways with early oncology and palliative care input to ensure appropriate care was given.

Against this background, the cancer patient journey not infrequently interfaces with multiple institutions and departments, and poses key challenges for patients, families and the evolving acute oncology services. In the patient population reviewed by NCEPOD, all of whom died within 30 days of receiving systemic anti-cancer therapy, 42% of them were admitted to a general medical service rather than to an oncology service. In addition 43% of all patients had either grade 3 or grade 4, life-threatening toxicity from their SACT recorded during their admission to hospital prior to their deaths. Of the NCEPOD population, 86% of patients were being treated with palliative intent and 50% of patients were on their second or subsequent line of SACT. It was notable that 15% of the NCEPOD study population, prior to their death, were admitted to a healthcare organization other than that which had actually delivered their chemotherapy, implying a lack of continuity of care. The findings suggest that factors in the deaths of these patients included toxicity from chemotherapy, often experienced by patients who were being treated with palliative intent. The admissions, sometimes to organisations other than those who were providing the SACT, and often to general medical services which were not specialized in oncology, might have resulted in some delay or inappropriate provision of treatment. Acute oncology services are charged with improving the quality of care for this and other patient populations."

Irrespective of local hospital or network solutions, acute oncology is underpinned by a number of core principles that promote education, awareness and early access to specialist oncology teams. In these models early specialist review must be combined with strong leadership and innovative service developments that will improve the safety and quality of emergency cancer care.

The number and type of acute oncology emergency admissions is highly dependent on local service configuration. This reflects the role of an individual hospital trust as an acute district general hospital, a fully integrated cancer centre or a standalone cancer centre that lacks acute medical and surgical support. For each of these services, the core acute oncology principles remain the same; however, the models of care may appear very different.

Data on acute oncology patterns and workload remain sparse. In 2006/07 there were 273 000 emergency admissions with a diagnosis of cancer, representing a 30% increase from 1997/98.[2] This is roughly equivalent to 750 emergency admissions each day across England, so that a typical trust may have five emergency admissions with cancer per day (two under general medicine, one under general surgery, one under oncology/haematology and one under 'other'). Unplanned cancer admissions may happen several times for the same patient. Average length of stay for inpatient cancer admissions between regions varied from 5.1 to 10.1 days in 2008/09. If every region had the same length of stay as the average in regions in the best performing quartile, even with no reduction in admissions, 566 000 bed-days could be saved, equivalent to £113 million each year.[1]

A one-day snapshot of inpatients at a combined acute university hospital trust and cancer centre identified that cancer patients accounted for 19% of all inpatients and that 57% of these had a known diagnosis of cancer.[4] Patients admitted under oncology had a shorter length of stay than those admitted under general medicine or general surgery (median 7 vs 18 days).

At the wider network level, the seven Acute Oncology Teams (AOTs) in the Merseyside and Cheshire Cancer Network (MCCN) reviewed 3031 cases following their first year of establishment, with monthly referral rates reaching a plateau after six months of inception.[5] The acute oncology type is shown in Tables 1.1 and 1.2. Patients admitted with complications of cancer at a time of disease progression represent the majority, with lung cancer the most frequent primary site. Emergency presentation of malignancy of undefined primary origin (MUO) accounted for 290 'type 1' acute oncology episodes.

Data collected prospectively by the AOTs revealed an average length of stay for the MCCN network as a whole to be 9.7 days. Comparing present average length of stay with baseline average on 2005/6 (12.8 days) shows a reduction of 3.1 days for cancer patients admitted to hospital since the network-wide AOS was implemented. This equates to a total number of 9014 bed-days saved.

Table 1.1 Acute oncology subtypes across Merseyside and Cheshire Cancer Network

AO Trust	Type 1 (new cancer)		Type 2 (chemo/ radiation comps <6wks)		Type 3 (know cancer complications)		Other		Not recorded		Total N
	N	%	N	%	N	%	N	%	N	%	
1	100	13%	154	21%	482	65%	0	0.0%	6	0.8%	742
2	130	23%	203	35%	239	42%	0	0.0%	2	0.3%	574
3	92	16%	248	43%	241	41%	0	0.0%	1	0.2%	582
4	121	28%	74	17%	203	47%	7	1.6%	24	5.6%	429
5	33	20%	49	30%	79	49%	0	0.0%	1	0.6%	162
6	46	12%	125	33%	200	53%	1	0.3%	6	1.6%	378
7	42	26%	42	26%	80	48%	0	0%	0	0%	164
Total	**564**		**895**		**1524**		**8**		**40**		**3031**

Table 1.2 Acute oncology referrals – top four primary sites across Merseyside and Cheshire Cancer Network

Tumour site Group	Trust 1	Trust 2	Trust 3	Trust 4	Trust 5	Trust 6	Total
Lung	207	147	139	94	39	74	700
Breast	85	89	120	52	19	77	442
Colorectal	86	37	118	28	42	58	369
UKP	52	50	86	65	16	21	290

The clinical challenges identified by the NCEPOD report and the subsequent development of acute oncology services has, in the UK, resulted in determined activity to improve the quality of care available to the patients who are at risk. The National Health Service (NHS) has provided valuable funding for the development of these services. There is, at present, no single template for an AOS. The complexity of the provision of care, the diversity of hospital configurations and the way in which hospitals cooperate in their cancer networks is such that a single template would be unworkable. However, clear principles have been developed. We have therefore presented the options for patient care by describing the management that would be provided by three different acute oncology services in three different clinical cancer care networks. These bring out the approaches that have been used and demonstrate how the principles have been incorporated, or are in the process of being incorporated, into care patterns in the UK.

Model I: a standalone cancer centre (Merseyside and Cheshire Cancer Network)

The MCCN serves a population of 2.3 million with non-surgical oncology provision delivered via a 'hub-and-spoke' model coordinated from the Clatterbridge Cancer Centre (CCC), a single standalone cancer centre. The CCC functions as a tertiary referral service and manages approximately 10 000 new patient episodes and over 47 000 chemotherapy episodes per year. The CCC has no acute medical, surgical or intensive care facilities, and delivers the majority of elective chemotherapy via satellite chemotherapy day units situated in seven acute NHS trusts. New and follow-up patients are reviewed in defined outpatient clinic sessions that are held within the CCC and across the satellite cancer units. Subsequently, patients are prescribed chemotherapy according to a single network protocol book, and receive standardized patient information and a chemotherapy alert card. The model of care ensures that the majority of chemotherapy and outpatient services are delivered close to the patient's home via fixed outpatient sessions supported by visiting peripatetic medical and chemotherapy nursing staff. In this model, the CCC hosts a 24-hour chemotherapy triage service for all solid tumour patients who have received chemotherapy within the previous six weeks.

The MCCN has developed an acute hospital acute oncology model that consists of at least two visiting oncologists (one of whom is the acute oncology lead for the host trust), providing a 5-day service, equating to one programmed activity, equivalent to one half day of a consultant working time, of acute oncology support per day Monday to Friday. The oncologist also provides one or more site-specialized services at the same trust where they provide acute oncology support. The oncologists do not have their own beds, but are available in the hospital on a Monday-to-Friday basis to review patients as necessary. The lead acute oncology consultant also uses their acute oncology session to lead and develop the service, support cancer peer review and represent the acute trust at the level of the cancer network.

The AOT also consists of a minimum of one full-time equivalent oncology cancer nurse specialist, available Monday to Friday, 9 a.m. to 5 p.m. This is in addition to administrative support linked to the local cancer services department, which provides a focal point for referrals, clinical enquiries and data support pertaining to each patient episode referred to the AOT. The acute oncology nursing remit is pivotal to the running of the service and often represents the first point of contact for professional and patient enquires.

Emergency presentation of suspected cancer requires responsive pathways and access to fast-track clinics as a means of improving care and reducing emergency admissions. Acute oncology services are particularly well placed to coordinate management, either through direct access to acute oncology fast-track clinic slots (within established outpatient oncology sessions) or via early cross-referral pathways with existing site-specific multi-disciplinary teams (MDTs). In either scenario it is essential that AOTs work closely with expert site-specific MDTs to facilitate investigation, speedy diagnosis and appropriate treatment. In the context of the cited MUO referral, local acute oncology services are developing direct GP referral capacity via new fast-track acute oncology slots within existing oncology outpatient clinics.

How might standalone cancer centre acute oncology services facilitate the ongoing management of these patients?

For **patient 1**, the request was identified within local district general hospital cancer services and triaged to acute oncology. The patient was contacted directly via telephone and received information and symptom management with acute oncology nursing support. Subsequently, the patient was reviewed in the outpatient department by the AOT within five days of referral, thus reducing the risk of inappropriate site-specific referral or an emergency admission. Focused investigation, including prostate-specific antigen (PSA), confirmed a diagnosis of metastatic prostatic carcinoma and the patient was transferred to the uro-oncology team for ongoing management.

For **patient 2**, central chemotherapy triage directed the patient to their local emergency department (ED) and alerted local AO services via email. Acute oncology education and pathway development can ensure that patients presenting with known complications of chemotherapy are triaged and managed along defined inpatient pathways. The development of local acute oncology pathways with ED and haematology services ensured the patient received expert timely care at the point of admission and subsequent triage to a specialist haematology ward environment. Ongoing review within 24 working hours by AOTs ensured optimal communication with the treating team at the cancer centre, liaison with central cytotoxic pharmacy, provision of patient information and support, and the development of risk-adapted early discharge policies.

For **patient 3**, the finding of metastatic cancer following a CT scan triggered an immediate acute oncology referral. This was facilitated by an increasing awareness of acute oncology services, and underpinned by a radiology flagging policy and acute oncology pathways that are placed on the hospital intranet. The patient was admitted to a general medical ward but reviewed within 24 hours by a member of the acute oncology team. In view of the patient's poor performance status, further investigations were cancelled, urgent review by the hospital palliative care team was undertaken and the case and imaging were reviewed at the weekly acute oncology MDT.

Model II: a comprehensive cancer centre (Yorkshire Cancer Network)

The Yorkshire Cancer Network (YCN) serves a population of approximately 2.6 million within the Yorkshire and Humber Strategic Health Authority. Non-surgical oncology provision is delivered via a cancer centre – the St James's Institute of Oncology (SJIO) – based in Leeds Teaching Hospitals Trust, and six additional hospital trusts providing cancer unit services with resident medical oncologists in the surrounding region. The cancer centre at Leeds functions both to provide local services for the people of Leeds and as a tertiary referral service for the YCN providing specialist cancer services for intermediate and rare cancers. The SJIO manages approximately 8000 new referrals per year, with 4500 patients receiving treatment and in excess of 22 000 chemotherapy episodes. The SJIO is a purpose-built cancer wing within a large teaching hospital providing emergency, acute medical, surgical and intensive care facilities. It also delivers all elective cancer treatment (chemotherapy and radiotherapy) within the centre. Patients living in the rest of the network are generally seen and treated by resident oncologists in the additional cancer units so that treatment is delivered close to the patient's home wherever possible. For the purpose of this chapter, further management will be discussed assuming the patients are, or will be, treated in the cancer centre.

All patients receiving treatment for cancer at SJIO are given a contact card (credit card-sized) with the appropriate numbers to call if they develop a complication of their cancer or treatment. This is a 24-hour triage service that is designed for all patients who have received treatment within the previous six weeks. If a patient calls, appropriate triage is carried out over the phone and a decision made whether or not the patient requires admission. Within SJIO there is a 4-bed assessment unit staffed by nurse practitioners and junior doctors designed for assessment of such patients, and an acute admissions ward for direct admission where appropriate. Very few patients attend the ED routinely in the model of care at SJIO, but good links are established to enable direct admission to acute oncology from the ED when necessary.

Within the YCN, acute oncology models are being developed independently in all the trusts in the network since resident medical oncologists exist locally in all trusts. The acute oncology model being developed at Leeds will consist of 20 programmed activities (PAs) of consultant time which is the equivalent of two full time consultants, providing a five-day service with the equivalent of around two PAs of support per day, Monday to Friday. Patients admitted to the Leeds hospitals with a suspected metastatic cancer will be referred to the AOS, and all patients are reviewed within 24 hours of referral to assist with appropriate choice of investigations, ongoing symptom management and other specialist advice.

How might comprehensive cancer centre acute oncology services facilitate the ongoing management of these patients?

Patients who present with suspected metastatic MUO, as illustrated in **patient 1**, are currently managed via existing two-week cancer referral pathways to defined cancer site-specific teams and managed in the outpatient setting where possible. Once the acute oncology MUO/cancer of unknown primary (CUP) service is fully developed and available, the GP might instead make a direct fast-track outpatient referral to the AOS if the patient is ambulatory and can be managed in the outpatient setting. The MUO/CUP team could then carry out the initial work-up and investigation of the patient, including assessing whether urgent oncological intervention is required, but also undertaking well informed discussion about potential diagnoses. Once the patient had been fully investigated and a confirmed site-specific diagnosis of metastatic prostate cancer determined, the patient would be referred quickly and appropriately to the urological cancer team to take over and continue the patient's care.

For patients who are already identified as cancer patients and being managed by cancer services in Leeds within the SJIO, there are already well established pathways for management of complications of their cancer or treatment, such as the febrile neutropenia seen in **patient 2**. If patients are unwell and require assessment or admission to hospital whilst on treatment they are reviewed on the assessment unit, or admitted to the acute admissions ward within SJIO and managed by an on-call team initially, but the following morning their care will be handed over to the site-specific team which is already responsible for the delivery of their treatment. This site-specific team will continue to provide their care whilst they are an inpatient within the oncology service in SJIO.

Suspected newly diagnosed cancer patients who require admission due to ill health or for inpatient investigation are currently managed by admission to the appropriate acute medical or surgical speciality, with input from oncology as requested. With the introduction of an AOS at Leeds, oncology involvement in the management of such patients will happen much earlier in the patient's pathway. In the case of **patient 3** above, presenting acutely to the ED with a suspected underlying cancer diagnosis, early referral through to the AOT will not only allow for early specialist input regarding appropriate investigation, management and referral to the correct MDT, but will also help facilitate early discharge from hospital with appropriate support and follow-up.

Model III: An acute cancer unit model (Whittington Health)

In April 2011, the Whittington Hospital NHS Trust joined up with the NHS Haringey and Islington community health services to form an integrated care organization, called Whittington Health (WH). This alliance has enabled local NHS service providers to work together to deliver patient care. It brings services and clinicians closer together, ensuring that care is more centred on the needs of local people and allows patients to navigate more easily between the services that they need. This new organization of care has allowed traditional barriers to be overcome, thus optimizing care pathway for patients.

In April 2012 the old cancer networks of North Central and North East London merged to form London Cancer: an integrated cancer system (ICS). The ICS serves a population of 3.5 million across North London and West Essex. Care for specialist tumour types will be delivered through pathway boards with representation from each of the nine trusts that comprise the ICS. Acute oncology services across the ICS will be addressed via an expert reference group. Building on the AOS developed at the Whittington Hospital NHS Trust cancer unit, fast-track pathways for GPs have been established as well as pathways developed for acute oncology admissions via the ED.

Whittington Health has developed an acute oncology model that consists of a stand-alone Consultant Medical Oncologist sub-specializing in lung and gastrointestinal cancers, speciality doctor, in oncology, haematology consultant and two oncology clinical nurse specialists, providing a comprehensive 5-day service. The Consultant Medical Oncologist is responsible for consultancy for all inpatients admitted to a designated medical ward with an oncology-related admission. Clear admission guidelines have been approved to ensure appropriate patients are admitted under the care of the consultant. In addition, the AOT offers daily review of all acute oncology admissions in outlying wards and those housed in the medical admissions unit. The Consultant Medical Oncologist was also appointed as Lead Cancer Clinician and so used their sessions to lead and further develop the AOS, support cancer peer review, and represent the acute trust at cancer network level. The Consultant Medical Oncologist chaired the network acute oncology group for two years from 2010.

The referral pathways were built into existing electronic order communications systems so are familiar to users, are cost neutral, and have inbuilt audit trails and data collection capacity owned and managed by the existing information technology (IT) team. This has also reduced the need for specific administrative support for the AOS, as all relevant clinical data can be accessed via the electronic order communications system where referrals are held on each patient. Additional acute oncology administrative support is provided by two oncology secretaries, who will type letters, make appointments and retrieve archived correspondence, as well as provide a telephone contact for any administrative query from a patient or healthcare professional.

How might the acute cancer centre services facilitate ongoing management of these patients?

For **patient 1**, the GP could make a direct fast-track acute oncology outpatient referral if the patient is ambulatory. This could not only avoid an unnecessary admission or presentation via the ED, but can enable prompt assessment by the expert AOT. The role of the AOT here is twofold: firstly, urgent assessment to determine if prompt oncological intervention is indicated, and secondly to communicate empathically and knowledgeably about the overall situation if this is a first presentation of a previously undiagnosed cancer. If the patient has any evidence of neurological impairment which threatens mobility the patient can be referred to the ED or the duty medical registrar, who will alert the malignant spinal cord coordinator (MSCC) within the AOT. A pathway exists that is approved by the cancer network to ensure prompt diagnosis and access to neurosurgery if indicated. All trusts have on-site chemotherapy facilities if urgent chemotherapy is the treatment of choice, and designated centres for radiotherapy have been approved. Data collected and collated from the NCIN consistently show that the prognosis and outcomes for all solid tumour cancer types that present for the first time via the ED is significantly worse than for those that present through the traditional two-week wait or urgent outpatient referrals. Acute oncology has a key role in ensuring appropriateness of further investigation, especially if the patient is of poor performance status or has multiple comorbidities.

In the second scenario, where **patient 2** is receiving a systemic anticancer chemotherapy regimen with a greater than 20% chance of febrile neutropenia, there would be an alert attached to the patient's ED file as well as a patient-specific protocol held by the relevant regional ambulance service (the London Ambulance Service in this case). In this way, as soon as a call is made to the emergency services from the patient's home an ambulance will be triggered to provide a blue-light service to ensure the patient is rapidly assessed and resuscitated if necessary before arrival in the ED. The ambulance service will also call ahead to prepare the ED team to expect a patient with suspected febrile neutropenia. This protocol has optimized the delivery of systemic antibiotics to patients within 60 minutes of arrival to the ED.

With **patient 3** the admitting medical team would have requested an inpatient AOS assessment and referred the case for discussion at the weekly MUO MDT. A separate radiology alert would have been triggered at the time of preparing the report of the CT scan. This ensures that if admitting teams delay referral to the AOS an e-mail alert is sent to a confidential and specific e-mail address by the reporting consultant radiologist.

Once assessed by the AOT within 24 hours of referral, the patient's fitness and personal wishes regarding further interventions would have been established. In view of her poor performance status, invasive investigations such as liver biopsy would not have changed her management so would not be routinely ordered. The priority for this lady's care would be to optimize symptom control and agree on the preferred place of care. Further management would be undertaken with the community palliative care team on discharge.

A follow-up alert would be placed on her ED record to direct appropriate investigations and care should she present again in the future.

Conclusion

Solutions and options for acute oncology require effective leadership and a clear understanding of cancer patient pathways within cancer networks and also within individual hospital trusts. The models described above exist within a complex and diverse cancer service configuration, but all share the common themes of triage, cancer alerts, early specialist review and defined inpatient pathways. These are all areas that have been highlighted by the NHS Improvement Transforming Inpatient Care programme.[6]

Acute oncology services are applying these principles to improve the management of patients admitted to hospital. In future it should be possible to work closely with colleagues in primary care to extend these principles to identify more precisely those patients who require admission and those who may be managed safely in the community. Improvements remain possible in the investigation of patients with suspected cancer, both to arrive more rapidly at an accurate diagnosis and to promptly ensure referral to the appropriate specialist teams. Early in a patient's journey we must take account of their fitness and their wishes about appropriate investigations and subsequent interventions.

Further reading

1 National Audit Office. *Department of Health: Delivering the Cancer Reform Strategy*. Norwich: TSO; Nov 2010. HC568, Session 2010–11. 44pp.

2 Mort D, Lansdown M, Smith N, Protopapa K, Mason M. *For better, for worse? A review of the care of patients who died within 30 days of receiving systemic anti-cancer therapy*. London: National Confidential Enquiry into Patient Outcome and Death (NCEPOD); Nov 2008. 150pp.

3 National Chemotherapy Advisory Group. *Chemotherapy Services in England: Ensuring quality and safety*. London: Department of Health; 21 Aug 2009. 70pp.

4 Mansour D, Simcock R, Gilbert DC. Acute oncology service: assessing the need and its implications. *Clin Oncol (R Coll Radiol)* 2011; **23**: 168-173.

5 Smith R, Marshall E, Neville-Webbe H, Andrews J, Hayes J. Innovation: When the big 'C' stands for creativity. *Health Serv J* 2012; **122**: 26-27.

6 NHS Improvement [Internet]. Transforming Inpatient Care. The Winning Principles. Leicester: NHS Improvement; c.2009. Available from: www.improvement.nhs.uk/cancer/inpatients/winningprinciples.html

02 Nursing Developments in Acute Oncology

Jeanette Ribton, Kathryn Oddy

Case History

A 72-year-old woman with increasing back pain attended a planned appointment in the rheumatology outpatient department on a Friday morning. A previously requested CT scan identified multiple bone metastases, and the rheumatology specialist registrar advised direct admission via the acute medical unit for further investigation and management. The admissions unit referred the patient to the acute oncology service.

How do acute oncology nursing services differ between district general hospitals and cancer centres?

How would your service respond to this patient?

How would you develop the nursing role in acute oncology?

Background

Acute oncology nursing: a district general hospital perspective

St Helens and Knowsley Teaching Hospitals NHS Trust (SHK) is a district general hospital working in partnership with Clatterbridge Cancer Centre (CCC) providing local delivery of care to patients receiving chemotherapy for solid tumours in the Merseyside and Cheshire area.

Historically, in many district general hospitals (DGH) oncology services are delivered by a limited number of oncology outpatient department and chemotherapy clinics. Inpatients requiring oncology assessment were reviewed on an *ad hoc* basis depend on the availability of oncology consultants and their awareness of the patient's admission. Treatment by site-specific cancer nurse specialists also fell into the same model. This often resulted in avoidable admission and delayed management, with frustration for both the patient and the ward team. The National Confidential Enquiry into Patient Outcome and Death (NCEPOD)[1] and the National Chemotherapy Advisory Group (NCAG)[2] recognized that rapid management of acute oncology conditions was often poor, and recommended service improvement and implementation of acute oncology teams.

Acute oncology nursing in a DGH is a unique and flexible role that provides the opportunity to develop a service driven by the needs of the local organization to support patients and generalist physicians in primary and secondary care.

The patient described above required multidisciplinary input and coordination, which previously was only achieved following hospital admission. In this instance, the patient was referred to oncology at the point of admission and reviewed the same day by the acute oncology cancer nurse specialist, who:

- discussed the CT findings with the patient and her family
- discovered that the patient wanted to go home – she was celebrating her grandson's 18th birthday and her husband's 70th birthday that weekend
- facilitated palliative care referral for assessment the same day
- facilitated district nurse referral for pain management over the weekend
- discharged the patient home safely that same day
- organized an oncology outpatient clinic for the following Monday.

The patient attended her family gatherings and attended clinic on the Monday with her family to discuss her future management.

This case illustrates effective collaboration between multiple departments and professionals. The family were supported in taking some control, and, most importantly, the patient attended two very important family gatherings. In the past this lady would have remained in hospital awaiting review by a consultant oncologist prior to any decision making. In fact, she was reviewed by a consultant oncologist in the outpatient setting more rapidly than if she had remained on the ward. This was possible as the acute oncology nursing focus is to streamline and improve patient pathways by overcoming barriers and understanding the whole patient pathway and experience.

Acute oncology nursing: a cancer centre perspective

The St James's Institute of Oncology (SJIO) is a large cancer centre based within Leeds Teaching Hospitals Trust which provides local delivery of care to patients living in Leeds and surrounding areas for all cancers, and acts as a tertiary referral centre for patients with rare cancers.

The SJIO responded to the challenge of acute oncology through a significant reconfiguration of the pathways and staff who care for those cancer patients presenting as an acute admission to the cancer centre. The reconfiguration of acute oncology services with the creation of a dedicated cancer acute admissions ward and cancer acute assessment unit took place, and a senior nurse coordinator was appointed to actively manage the available bed base and ensure projected dates of discharge are defined on all patients on admission. To try to improve the management of acute oncology problems, two senior acute oncology nurse practitioners were also appointed to triage admissions and commence appropriate investigation and management according to defined protocols.

In addition to the above, consultants with time in their schedule to dedicate to acute oncology have been, or are in the process of being, appointed. Together with the support of an advanced nurse practitioner and the two senior nurse practitioners, the consultants will be responsible for developing the outreach acute oncology service as well as managing the Acute Assessment Unit.

The nursing role within SJIO acute oncology is vital to the efficient and effective running of the service. Patients will be referred to the Acute Oncology Team (AOT) through a single route via either faxed referral form or a telephone referral. These referrals will be triaged daily by the acute oncology nurse practitioners and the urgency of review determined. Review of the patients will take place by the appropriate AOT member within 24 hours of referral, often by the nurse practitioners initially, and appropriate advice and support given.

Despite the difference in acute oncology staffing models between the DGH and the cancer centre, the principles of care are the same. The patient in this case would have been managed in the same way – the acute oncology nurses reviewing the patient on the medical ward and facilitating early discharge from hospital with appropriate support and outpatient follow-up.

Recent Developments

Developing the nursing role

Both the acute oncology nurse practitioners in the cancer centre and the GH will develop the same clinical skills and will need to provide expert oncological advice, not only to acute specialties but also the more junior nursing colleagues in oncology/haematology itself.

The acute oncology service is a multidisciplinary team approach and the acute oncology nurse is the face to both patients and non-oncology professionals of acute oncology, and crucial to the success of the service and peer review. Peer review measures direct the future for acute oncology with an emphasis on both clinical and patient outcomes.[3] The measures set clear objectives aimed at improving the care for people with cancer and their families. Some of the targets are challenging but nevertheless necessary to improve the quality and effectiveness of care. The key themes and policy documents are highlighted in Table 2.1.

Table 2.1 Peer review themes and policy documents
Key peer review themes
1. Structure and function of the service
2. Coordination of care pathways
3. Patient experience
4. Clinical outcomes/indicators
The three key policies required are:
1. Operational policy
2. Annual report
3. Work plan

Some key points to help develop the acute oncology service

Developing AO nurses' clinical skill set

- Clinical skills such as examinations, diagnostics, nurse prescribing
- Advanced communication skills
- Leadership skills
- Acute oncology module
- Knowledge of the UK Oncology Nursing Society (UKONS) 'Oncology/Haematology 24 Hour Triage Rapid Assessment and Access Tool Kit'.[4]

Referral systems

Ease of access for advice is essential. Include out of hours advice (maybe from the cancer centre).

Job plans

Ideally, two acute oncology nurses are required to ensure cross-cover and the successful implementation of acute oncology nursing. In the DGH model, 50% of each nurse's time is expected to be dedicated to managing the inpatient services. An illustrative job plan is shown in Table 2.2.

Table 2.2 District general hospital acute oncology nursing job plan

Monday	Tuesday	Wednesday	Thursday	Friday
Mini MDT (within the chemo unit) to discuss inpatients Outpatient clinic	Inpatient visits	Inpatient visits Palliative care MDT	Outpatient clinic AOT MDT	Inpatient visits
Inpatient visits	Audit/service development Messages/ telephone support	Chemotherapy unit support	Inpatient visits Messages/ telephone support	Messages/telephone clinic CPD

Ensure you allow time for administration and service development to strategically plan the future service and develop pathways. AOT, acute oncology team; CPD, continuous professional development; MDT, multi-disciplinary team

Engaging with key professionals and departments

Coordination of patient care and awareness of acute oncology services requires a high level of engagement with key departments within the hospital (Table 2.3).

Support and mentorship from your oncology team

Weekly multidisciplinary team (MDT) meeting: developing the team is important to ensure sustainability and service development. The AOT should be a multiprofessional group with an active MDT. The MDT coordinator role is invaluable in supporting the nurses to collate information/data and track patients' investigations and appointments following discharge. The MDT ensures cancer patients requiring acute oncology review have optimal management of their treatment or cancer-related complications, with timely discharge and onward referral to oncology/palliative care services as needed.

Table 2.3 Key departmental relationships with Acute Oncology

Emergency dept/ AMU daily visits/ ward visits	Early referral, assessment and management plan Advice on necessary/unnecessary investigations Plan for discharge/fast access to outpatient clinics Timely and appropriate referral to other specialists Education to ward staff Pathway development Communication Influence management and service development	
	Induction training is necessary for:	A&E staff – medical staff and senior nurses (Band 6) or above
		AMU staff – medical staff and senior nurses (Band 6) nurse or above
		Encourage link nurses to help to sustain the service
Chemotherapy unit & triage	Proactive assessment of unwell patients to avoid admission Liaison regarding the management for inpatients and future care	
Site-specific	Highlight specific wards to help manage specific complications. This will help to develop and streamline pathways and	
	ensure expert care, e.g.:	Haematology (neutropenic sepsis) Gastro (chemotherapy-induced diarrhoea)
Palliative Care Team	Some patients may require joint visits with AO	

Table 2.4 An illustrative multidisciplinary team (MDT)

Consultant medical oncology
Consultant clinical oncology
Consultant radiologist
Consultant palliative care
Consultant pathologist (attends on a need basis only)
Clinical nurse specialists (×2)
MDT coordinator
Secretary (does not need to attend)

Driving the acute oncology service forward

Measuring the impact of your acute oncology service – aiming to measure your values, outcomes and successes – will provide evidence to maintain and grow the service. Ask the cancer network to help develop an audit tool and collate the data. The dataset includes: demographics, date of admission, diagnosis, chemotherapy and last cycle (if applicable),

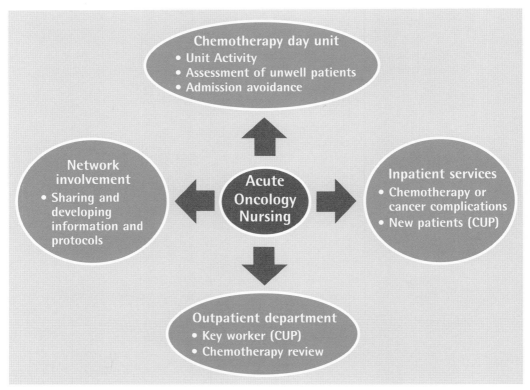

Figure 2.1 Acute oncology nursing roles.

referral method, time to acute oncology review, admitting ward, reason for admission, and a summary.

Create an acute oncology nursing forum within your cancer network to share best practice, develop pathways and provide peer support. This will help to standardize clinical practice regionally.

Disseminating information regularly to core group members and steering group members will increase your chances of success. Resistance is common following a change so be prepared to reiterate your plans to the wider trust regularly.[5]

Conclusion

 Acute oncology models may differ from trust to trust and between networks depending on the set up; however, the ultimate objectives remain the same. The patient is at the heart of any healthcare service, therefore it is vital that healthcare professionals understand the patient's experience and continually improve their service.

Acute oncology nursing is complex as it covers a wide arena of symptoms, different cancers and patients who often require a multitude of interventions and procedures. Acute oncology nurses have an opportunity to take cancer nursing forward, improving patient care and services. Acute oncology nurses are also ideally placed to lead in the management of oncology patients within secondary care. In addition, the future of acute oncology nursing represents an opportunity to develop a structure that avoids hospital admission and promotes patient ambulatory care. Coordination of care and communication are key to evolving clinical practice.

Further reading

1 Mort D, Lansdown M, Smith N, Protopapa K, Mason M. *For better, for worse? A review of the care of patients who died within 30 days of receiving systemic anti-cancer therapy.* London: National Confidential Enquiry into Patient Outcome and Death (NCEPOD); Nov 2008. 150pp.

2 National Chemotherapy Advisory Group. *Chemotherapy Services in England: Ensuring quality and safety.* London: Department of Health; 21 Aug 2009. 70pp.

3 National Cancer Peer Review-National Cancer Action Team. *Acute Oncology Measures.* London: Department of Health; 7 Apr 2011. 50pp.

4 Jones PJ, *et al.*, UKONS, GMCN. *Oncology/Haematology 24 Hour Triage Rapid Assessment and Access Tool Kit.* Published by UK Oncology Nursing Society; Oct 2010. 28pp. c.2010 P.Jones, UKONS Central West Chemotherapy Nurses Group and The Greater Midlands Cancer Network.

5 Cameron E, Green M. *Making Sense of Change Management.* 2nd ed. London: Kogan Page; 2009.

03 Cancer of Unknown Primary (CUP)

Richard Osborne

Case History

A 68-year-old man attended the emergency department at the weekend with sudden onset of pain in his right arm after minor trauma. He had a number of other non-specific symptoms including general malaise and weight loss. X-rays revealed an undisplaced pathological fracture of the right humerus and other bone metastases. A set of routine blood tests was requested, though not reviewed. The patient was discharged home the same day with a sling by a junior member of the orthopaedic team who also arranged referral to a multidisciplinary team (MDT).

How can this patient's cancer be categorized for appropriate referral and ongoing care?

What organizational shortcomings might exist that would prevent this patient receiving optimal care?

What system of immediate care should established for patients such as this?

How should the subsequent care of patients on the MUO/CUP spectrum be organized (see Table 3.1)?

How has the paradigm for treatment of CUP changed recently?

Background

How should this patient's cancer be categorized for appropriate referral and ongoing care?

This patient provides an example of a common dilemma. He almost certainly has cancer, but in current practice there is uncertainty about how he should be further investigated, who should be responsible for this task, and who should coordinate delivery of services for his ancillary needs of information, support and symptom control.

He has features of metastatic bone disease, but has not undergone any subsequent tests designed to characterize the disease more precisely. The differential diagnosis is broad, ranging from a primary bone tumour (with metastases), to myeloma, to the most common scenario of bone metastases from a recognized primary such as kidney, stomach or lung. Ultimately, if carcinoma is confirmed but all other investigations are completed without a primary site being identified, the patient would be classified as having cancer of unknown primary (CUP). In terms of initial care, a similar dilemma is frequently encountered when patients present *de novo* with other common manifestations of metastatic cancer, such as malignant liver disease, malignant ascites, malignant pleural effusions, brain metastases, malignant nodes or other malignant masses.

One factor which has blocked developments in this setting is the lack of specific language to delineate the clinical entity, and hence to allow appropriate focus on service development. This has been rectified recently by standard definitions provided in the NICE Clinical Guideline for 'Metastatic malignant disease of unknown primary origin (CG104)', summarized in Table 3.1.[1]

Table 3.1 Definitions following NICE Clinical Guidelines CG104.
Malignancy of undefined primary origin (MUO) Metastatic malignancy identified on the basis of a limited number of tests, without an obvious primary site, before comprehensive investigation.
Provisional carcinoma of unknown primary origin (provisional CUP, pCUP) Metastatic epithelial or neuroendocrine malignancy identified on the basis of histology or cytology, with no primary site detected despite a selected initial screen of investigations, before specialist review and possible further specialized investigations.
Confirmed carcinoma of unknown primary origin (confirmed CUP, cCUP) Metastatic epithelial or neuroendocrine malignancy identified on the basis of final histology, with no primary site detected despite a selected initial screen of investigations, specialist review, and further specialized investigations as appropriate.

The concept of metastatic malignancy of undefined primary origin (metastatic MUO) is now embedded among acute oncology practitioners, with beneficial consequences. It is becoming possible to collect reliable data on incidence rate, allowing workforce planning. Agreement on the existence of MUO and its wide recognition should now permit appropriate management to be introduced in a more timely and uniform fashion.

What organizational shortcomings might exist that would prevent a patient with MUO receiving optimal care?

Although cancer services for patients with an established primary site are well developed, this system of care does not efficiently serve those in whom the origin of metastatic cancer is unknown. The relatively rigid and compartmentalized nature of site-specific cancer management has actually resulted in a deterioration in skills and facilities for generic diagnosis and care.

Compared with a patient in whom a site-specific cancer diagnosis is clear, the patient with MUO faces numerous significant, *immediate* problems:

- The lack of an explicit, efficient, formal system to manage the initial diagnostic phase
- Inadequate information about their illness
- Uncertainty about the nature and organization of clinical plans
- Insufficient symptom control and delayed access to specialist palliative care
- No cancer nurse specialist support
- Referral to an inappropriate site-specific cancer team using a process which does not provide necessary information for decision making, leading to delays in investigation and treatment.

Additionally, as seen with the patient described above, the current vogue for ambulatory care and rapid discharge means that formal arrangements for management of outstanding clinical problems are often neglected. In this case, the lack of continuity of care meant that serious problems due to metastatic malignancy involving bones (e.g. hypercalcaemia, uncontrolled pain, other fractures, spinal cord compression, myeloma complications) could have been present or developed subsequently, leading to additional yet avoidable morbidity.

The list of deficiencies in current care arrangements can be further expanded when other clinical scenarios are considered. For MUO patients identified in primary care there are no specific referral guidelines to assist timely expert assessment. Currently, oncological and palliative care advice is only accessed after significant delay, with adverse consequences in terms of speed and quality of decision making, efficiency (in terms of length of stay) and patient satisfaction. The latter point warrants reinforcement. The debilitating uncertainty experienced by patients and carers is a direct consequence of a lack of specialist services in this area, meaning the development of dedicated expert care for this very common scenario is an urgent priority.

The main purpose of this chapter is therefore to provide guidance on the organization of services for optimal acute care of MUO and CUP, rather than to act as a didactic tool for investigation and management of the specific clinical problems seen in this group. Information about modern strategies for investigation of MUO and treatment for common acute complications of malignant disease is easily found elsewhere.[1-4]

Recent Developments

What system of immediate care should be established for patients with MUO?

The appropriate organization of care for patients with MUO/CUP is defined in detail in the National Cancer Peer Review Programme Manual for Cancer Services Cancer of Unknown Primary Measures.[5] The key principle is that the NICE CUP Guideline:

> "… *recognizes the validity for MUO/CUP of the same basic service infrastructure which underpins that for site specific cancers, as outlined in the various Improving Outcomes Guidance publications and The Manual for Cancer Services. That is, multidisciplinary teams, network site specific groups, various related hospital services and the cancer network.*"

Accordingly, the main components required are:

1. *A "CUP Team" to advise on, and supervise appropriate investigation and subsequent management, according to the guidelines in NICE CG104.*[1]

   The team should comprise a consultant oncologist with expertise in MUO/CUP, a palliative medicine consultant, and a designated cancer nurse specialist. The CUP team will, with other colleagues in radiology and pathology, along with necessary administrative support, undertake traditional MDT functions. The team will meet weekly to review all new patients and to ensure the necessary input is available to deliver comprehensive care for each individual.

   An important concept is that the newly presenting patient with MUO will usually remain under the care of the admitting (non-oncology) consultant initially, with the

CUP team exercising an advisory role. This arrangement is necessary where patients are admitted to hospitals without resident oncologists or oncology beds.

2. *A system for rapid review of inpatients, or access to rapid, dedicated outpatient specialist oncologist assessment when MUO is diagnosed but admission is not required.*
   The necessity for prompt expert oncological advice, attention to symptomatic needs, and holistic support cannot be overemphasized. Equally, with this new approach, the ability to enter a generic process for investigation is expected to significantly benefit patients who would otherwise spend unacceptable amounts of time being investigated inappropriately by site-specific clinicians. It is important to recognize that these developments place novel demands on some oncologists whose proficiency in front-line diagnosis may not be fully developed. It is anticipated that the emergence of acute oncology as a subspecialty in oncology will largely overcome this problem.

3. *A full range of network-level functions (in common with the arrangements for known-site cancers) to underpin high quality care.*
   The CUP site-specific group (SSG) is essential to ensuring that this relatively common condition is accorded appropriate investment in terms of clinical and support resources. Additionally, for this neglected disease complex, the establishment and maintenance of explicit management guidelines and the delivery of ancillary functions, such as audit and research, is an obvious need.

   The precise arrangements for SSG working can be organized to suit the requirements of different networks. So long as the essential duties are conducted, it may be that some organizations will link the CUP SSG with another established SSG. Consideration should, however, be given to ensuring the highest-quality CUP service is delivered, in full compliance with the National Cancer Peer Review measures. There will be some configurations (for instance amalgamation within the acute oncology SSG) which may superficially appear logical, but which run the risk of neglecting aspects of CUP care (see below).

How should the subsequent care of patients on the MUO/CUP spectrum be organized?

Approaches developed for rapid problem solving in the acute phase after presentation with MUO must be complemented by suitable organization of care in the much longer phase of management and treatment that follows this. It is certainly reasonable to design and implement services for immediate care of newly presenting MUO within the context of emerging Acute Oncology Services (AOS), since the benefits arising from a rapid-response approach are well suited to the problems of this group. However, continuing care beyond the initial phase requires that 'disease-specific' structures, analogous to those for patients with known-site cancer, are put in place for those in whom a primary site is not rapidly identified.

For this sizeable cohort with 'provisional CUP', post-acute care remains compromised by:

- A lack of dedicated and specialist oncology expertise
- Uncertainty about appropriate advanced diagnostic tests, including the use of new technologies such as positron emission tomography (PET) and molecular profiling

- Lack of an overall organizational structure to ensure high-quality care through the whole patient journey
- Uncertainty about optimal treatment
- Lack of adequate epidemiology data
- No research organization.

Existing acute oncology models designed around the National Cancer Peer Review measures do not deliver these facilities. Recognition of the requirement for later, 'site-specific' arrangements for CUP is needed, analogous to those routinely provided for other major cancers. This has consequences when designing an overarching structure for MUO/CUP care. Simply concentrating on acute needs, based on an acute oncology SSG approach, cannot provide the necessary expertise and facilities to comprehensively address identified shortcomings in long-term care. Figure 3.1 demonstrates the distinction between overall MUO/CUP care and the acute oncology remit.

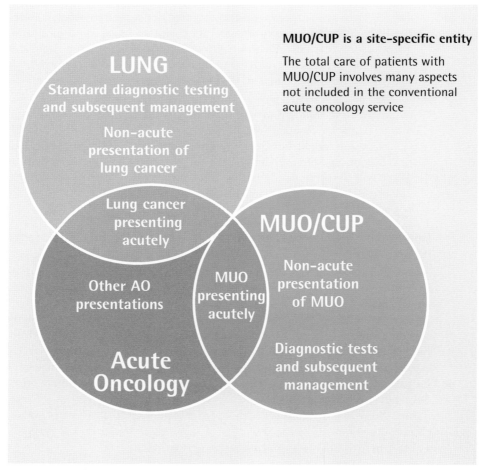

Figure 3.1 MUO/CUP is a site-specific entity. AO, acute oncology; CUP, carcinoma of unknown primary origin; MUO, malignancy of undefined primary origin.

How has the paradigm for treatment of CUP changed recently?

Having defined the desirable architecture for the comprehensive management of patients with MUO/CUP, it is important to consider actual therapeutic advances which can further improve care.

The past history of therapeutic nihilism surrounding CUP is, in a way, understandable, because the outcomes from treatment are very limited for the majority of patients. Lack of engagement with investigating and managing the condition has compounded the limitations of medical interventions such that this patient group has been uniquely disadvantaged.

This whole picture is now undergoing radical change. Oncologists are recognizing that management of MUO/CUP offers significant intellectual challenges which render the condition worthy of interest. The ability (and now the requirement)[5] to radically improve care through proper organization, aided by the introduction of AOS, means that this is a satisfying area of work. At the same time, tantalizing developments in treatment are emerging which have the ability to bring outcomes for CUP patients up towards the standards achieved in other common metastatic malignancies. Gene expression-based profiling (GEBP) has been investigated for many years in patients with confirmed CUP, and the weight of data now supports the potential of this approach to characterize patients as having a 'primary-like' genotype. When treated along site-specific lines, based on these results relating to tissue of origin, outcomes are beginning to match those expected in patients with known-site disease.[6,7] The policy of explicitly managing confirmed CUP patients along these lines is now achieving credence among experts in the field, though access to the necessary GEBP test is limited by cost at present.

Conclusions

In summary, it is anticipated that implementation of new organizational structures and services for MUO will radically improve many aspects of the patient journey. The growing acceptance of treatment of confirmed CUP along 'primary-like' lines will have a beneficial impact on the equally important outcomes of response and survival for this challenging condition.

Further reading

1   National Institute for Health and Clinical Excellence [Internet]. *Metastatic malignant disease of unknown primary origin (CG104)*. London: National Institute for Health and Care Excellence. c.2010. Available from: www.nice.org.uk/CG104

2   Armstrong A. Unknown primary: work-up and treatment. In: O'Donnell D, Leahy M, Marples M, Protheroe A, Selby P, eds. *Problem Solving in Oncology*.. Oxford: Clinical Publishing; 2008: p.27–31.

3   Baka S. Large abdominal mass. In: O'Donnell D, Leahy M, Marples M, Protheroe A, Selby P, eds. *Problem Solving in Oncology*. Oxford: Clinical Publishing; 2008: p.31–5.

4   Yeoh C. Ascites in an elderly patient. In: Edited by O'Donnell D, Leahy M, Marples M, Protheroe A, Selby P, eds. *Problem Solving in Oncology*. Oxford: Clinical Publishing; 2008: p.36–8.

5   National Cancer Peer Review Programme Manual for Cancer Services Cancer of Unknown Primary Measures. 2012. www.cquins.nhs.uk/xxxxx (full link to follow once Measures are published and uploaded in late October 2012.)

6   Hainsworth JD, Rubin MS, Spigel DR, *et al.* Molecular gene expression profiling to predict the tissue of origin and direct site specific therapy in patients with carcinoma of unknown primary site: A prospective trial of the Sarah Cannon Research Institute. *J Clin Oncol* 2013; **31**: 217–23.

7   Hainsworth JD, Schnabel CA, Erlander MG, *et al.* A retrospective study of treatment outcomes in patients with carcinoma of unknown primary site and a colorectal molecular profile. *Clin Colorectal Cancer* 2012; **11**: 112–8.

04 The Acute Cancer Patient in the Acute Medical Admitting Unit

Charlie Wilkinson, Alison Young

New approaches to acute oncology must build upon the experience of acute medicine

The challenge in providing a responsive service which meets the needs of acutely unwell patients admitted to hospital has been well studied within the arena of acute medicine. This chapter focuses on the key elements in acute hospital-based care in terms of facilities, policies, and how an acute oncology service (AOS) may complement pre-existing services to the benefit of patients.

Facilities: Background to the development of the acute medical unit

Traditionally, patients with a suspected medical illness requiring urgent hospital assessment would be directed to the ward of the general physician on call. They would expect to be cared for, regardless of medical condition, until their discharge or other outcome. However, over the past 25 years there has been considerable development in acute care in response to a variety of factors. These include an inexorable increase in acute admissions. Indeed emergency admissions via the emergency department (ED) or from primary care grew more rapidly in the UK than waiting list elective admissions between 2000 and 2001.[1] Coincident with rising admissions is the reduction of the acute hospital bed base by approximately a third over the past 25 years in the UK. Furthermore, patients themselves are becoming older, with increasingly complex and multiple comorbidities. Patients aged 85 years and over accounted for 4.8% of first attendances to English EDs in 2008/9, 62% of which were admitted.[2] Indeed, persons aged 85 years and above are almost 10 times more likely to be admitted to hospital than those aged 20–40 years.[2] Consequently, there have been changes in both the design and location of receiving facilities, and in the staffing skill mix and training for those working at the 'sharp end' to meet these challenges.

Patients admitted on the unselected medical take will include those with known or suspected cancer. Currently, these patients are often managed initially by staff whose primary area of expertise is not oncology. Hence, opportunity exists in which an AOS can work either alongside or within the acute medical service with defined care pathways to improve outcomes and patient satisfaction.

The Royal College of Physicians (RCP) began to address the challenge of acute medical care provision in 2000 with their report, *Acute Medicine: the physician's role*.[3] This encouraged the development of acute medical units (AMU) to focus admissions within a specific receiving area. This allowed the evolution of new models of consultant-led care delivery, development of nursing roles, and the establishment of professions with expertise working at the interface between community and hospital care. It is easy to see that, by applying improved care pathways in this area, patients can be directed to see 'the right person, in the right setting – first time', which was the title of the subsequent RCP report in 2007.[4] Therein, the vision for the AMU was developed in terms of its function and facility requirements. Although oncology patients are not addressed specifically, specialty 'in-reach' was seen as desirable.

The acute medical unit (AMU)

The concept of the AMU as defined by the RCP Acute Medicine Taskforce is of a 24-hour, 7-day week multidisciplinary dedicated facility acting as the focus for medical emergencies presenting to hospitals. It may also function as a facility for patients who have developed an acute medical illness whilst in hospital. It should ideally be located near to the hospital 'front door', within proximity to the ED. Also, easy access to critical care facilities and key diagnostic facilities is required. The recommended size should be roughly equivalent to the number of patients admitted in 24 hours plus 10%, though this will be influenced by organization of specific factors. These include bed base size and accessibility, short stay facility and community bed base availability.[4]

It is envisaged that an AMU would be capable of generating a discharge rate of between 30% and 40% of admissions directly, without unnecessary moves between wards within the hospital. A common configuration includes a short-stay facility in close proximity to the AMU, which is run by the same team of physicians to improve continuity of care. Patients identified early as expected to have an inpatient stay of less than 72 hours should be directed to short stay, in which patients are actively 'pulled' through the system. It is estimated that this should produce a combined discharge rate of up to 50% of admissions from both the AMU and short stay areas.

Facilities: Equipment and design requirements

In terms of equipment and design features, it is recommended that the AMU should have as a minimum the items shown in Table 4.1. Level 2 facilities within the AMU are desirable, but depend on the availability and proximity of high-dependency units within the organization.

Scheduled access seven days a week to diagnostics including GI endoscopy, echocardiography, diagnostic ultrasound, CT and MR imaging is recommended.

Access to a critical care outreach team is essential, with call-out algorithms based on the national early warning score (NEWS) or equivalent. Patients requiring specialist input should have access to specialty in-reach on the unit, or can be triaged to the appropriate bed base by a senior decision maker as early as possible.

Transfer of care planning should commence on initial assessment with accurate diagnostic coding and estimation of anticipated length of stay; the latter helps in identifying suitable short-stay patients and enables triage to specialty beds.

Ambulatory care and the virtual ward

There has been much interest in acute conditions which are amenable to innovative approaches that do not require inpatient management. These are termed ambulatory care-sensitive conditions (ACSCs). They can be broadly classified as chronic conditions in which effective management can prevent exacerbations, acute conditions in which intervention can prevent deterioration, and preventable conditions in which intervention can prevent illness. The acute medical conditions identified as ACSCs include

Table 4.1 Recommended facilities of an acute receiving medical unit (from ref. 4 and 5)

Core Accommodation

Trolleys, beds and chairs appropriate to the needs of patients, capable of flexing capacity to match
fluctuations in numbers and dependency of patients

Appropriate isolation facilities

Single-sex bay accommodation

Monitored beds capable of non-invasive ECG, blood pressure, and oxygen saturation monitoring

A high-dependency bed base with facilities for non-invasive ventilation (NIV) and continuous positive
airways pressure (CPAP) support in larger units unless provided adequately elsewhere

Support Facilities

Access to arterial blood gas analysis with a machine conforming to Good Laboratory Practice
regulations. Surviving sepsis recommendations support the requirement for a machine which can
measure lactate

A facility for assessing patients with mental health problems (confidential interview room)

Procedure room for intimate or invasive procedures

Resuscitation drugs and equipment

Facilities and space for physiotherapy and occupational therapy

Relatives' waiting area

Toilet and washing facilities for male and female patients

An appropriate area with chairs and trolley spaces which can be used by patients ready for discharge
or transfer who are awaiting transport

IT access (ideally wireless)

Equipment store

In-house pharmacy and medication treatment packs

Staff Facilities

A staff area or "operations room" for coordination of the acute medical team which also acts as a
coordination base out of hours for the Hospital at Night team

Administration and clerical space

Staff rest area, changing area and locker space

Dedicated teaching space

gastroenteritis, pyelonephritis, perforated or bleeding ulcer, cellulitis, epilepsy, angina,
iron deficiency anaemia, hypertension and nutritional deficiencies.[6] Low-risk pulmonary
embolism, pneumonia and deep vein thrombosis can also be treated in an ambulatory
fashion. It is likely that with involvement of an AOS a meaningful impact could be made
at an early stage, particularly if an ambulatory care area has agreed protocols for next day
imaging and review.

A high admission rate for ACSCs may indicate poor coordination between primary
and secondary care components of the local healthcare system. Therefore, much of acute
medicine development has focused on improving care pathways in this area. Some units
have developed innovative 'virtual wards' in which patients who remain ambulatory are
entered onto ward-based IT software systems and reviewed daily as though they are part

of the programmed inpatient ward round, but without admission to a hospital bed. Patient review is performed either by telephone, or direct review by recall to the assessment area for tests and clinical assessment as required.

Staffing, patient review provision and handover

An acute unit requires a strong multidisciplinary team with managerial, administrative and IT support. It is desirable for nursing staff to be encouraged to develop enhanced skills such as ECG recording, venepuncture and cannulation. There should be a nominated lead consultant and nurse who regularly perform clinical work on the unit. There should be a nominated shift leader on each shift who has an overview of all patients and the flow of patients through the unit, and who is responsible for liaison with bed managers.

Nurse-to-patient ratios required for the dependency of patients are normally 1:2 in high-dependency areas, 1:4 for patients who remain on mobile trolleys whilst awaiting decisions about admission or the location of admission, and 1:6 for patients in beds.

Other essential staff includes administrative and clerical cover (preferably 24 hours a day), community psychiatric nursing support, dedicated physiotherapy, occupational therapy and social worker input, dedicated pharmacy support, portering staff and cleaning staff, all of which facilitate rapid bed turnaround. Junior doctor staff ideally should be allocated to the acute unit for blocks of between two to four months in order to improve team building and develop competencies in acute assessment. This is seen as being superior to junior doctors dipping in and out of acute work when on call.

In October 2012 the RCP released *Acute Care Toolkit 4*, aimed at delivering a 12-hour, 7-day consultant presence on acute units.[7] Consultant staffing numbers should relate to the number of beds and admissions per 24 hours as shown in Table 4.2. Twice-daily consultant-led ward rounds are recommended, seven days a week, with rolling specialist registrar (SpR) reviews in between. All patients should be reviewed with a management plan devised within four hours of arrival. Table 4.2 also demonstrates the recommended numbers of consultant staff delivering care on an AMU per bed and admission numbers.

Table 4.2 Minimum number of consultants required on the acute unit (from ref. 4)

Approximate number of beds on admissions unit	Number of admissions per 24 hours	Number of consultants required on the unit 8am–8pm
≤30	≤25	1–1.5
30–50	25–44	1.5–2
51–70	45–60	2–3

Policies on the acute unit

The admissions unit should have agreed guidelines written into their operational policy which cover admission criteria and information given to patients (both condition-specific information), and documentation describing the unit and discharge process. The operational policy should also describe protocols for admission alternatives, the process for directing patients elsewhere if they are not admitted, tracking expected patients, investigations to be done prior to admission (if relevant), and how handover of clinical information should be done.

It is recommended that there is a standardized initial assessment by a triaging member of staff which includes early warning score calculation with appropriate escalation, initial brief history, ECG and pain score, all within 30 minutes of arrival. Observation frequency should be according to the early warning score, or every four hours as a minimum. A form template should be in use to enable a full clinical assessment and initiation of a management plan. A senior 'decision-maker' should review the admission within four hours of arrival.

Standardized evidence-based common presentation guidelines (standard operating policies) are recommended, which are developed and agreed with diagnostic services and relevant specialties. Other important considerations include medicines reconciliation, cannula care, catheter care and *Clostridium difficile* risk reduction.

The quality agenda

There is a drive to improve quality in acute care, which in the UK is led in part by the RCP as well as the Department of Health. The RCP *Acute Care Toolkit 2* recommends that early warning scores are widely used to assess the severity of illness, required on arrival as mentioned above for the standardized initial assessment.[8] Care bundles should be used for medical conditions in order to provide standardized comprehensive assessment of specified conditions, e.g. sepsis. Standardization of documentation for patient clerking, prescription of medication and intravenous fluids, and inpatient observation and fluid balance charts are also recommended. There is also a focus on handover and patient transfer out from the acute area.

Acute medicine and improving care of oncology patients: the acute oncology service (AOS)

It can be seen that a lot of development and improvement at the sharp end of acute hospital care is under way. How might the development of an AOS improve patient pathways for patients admitted acutely to the AMU with (a) new suspected cancer and (b) complications of existing cancer or cancer treatment?

Prior to the introduction of the concept of an AOS, patients admitted acutely via the AMU with what clinically appeared to be a suspected new diagnosis of cancer would be worked up to try to identify a clear diagnosis by general acute physicians. This often took place under inpatient status, necessitating lengthy hospital admissions due to an understandable reluctance to discharge such patients before results were back for fear of them getting lost in the system. This is less than ideal for several reasons: patients fit for discharge are kept in hospital, acute medical beds are being used where bed pressures constantly exist, and there is a lack of early specialist input for these patients. With the introduction of an AOS, a single point of contact service would be developed to allow early referral of patients admitted with suspected cancers. This would potentially reduce length of inpatient stay for this group of patients, help facilitate early specialist input, help facilitate appropriate investigation of patients and avoidance of over- or under-treatment, promote better communication between acute specialties, and lead to improved patient outcomes and satisfaction.

The development of an AOS will be of benefit to those patients presenting acutely to the AMU with complications of their cancer or cancer treatment. For hospital trusts with resident oncology services, a single point of contact for referring these patients to the AOS will again enable early specialist input and appropriate transfer of patients to oncology services. In hospital trusts where no resident oncology services exist, development of acute oncology management protocols (e.g. uncontrolled nausea and vomiting, uncontrolled mucositis, acute skin reactions, abdominal ascites, pleural effusion) that are readily available to all healthcare professionals, alongside the AOS referral service, will enable more appropriate and efficient management of such patients.

Further reading

1   NHS Information Centre [Internet]. *Hospital episode statistics. Headline figures 2010-2011.* www.hscic.gov.uk/hes

2   Blunt I, Bardsley M, Dixon J. Briefing. *Trends in emergency admissions in England 2004–2009: is greater efficiency breeding inefficiency?* London: The Nuffield Trust; Jul 2010. 12pp. Available from: www.nuffieldtrust.org.uk/publications/trends-emergency-admissions-england-2004-2009

3   Federation of Medical Royal Colleges. *Acute medicine: the physician's role. Proposals for the future. A working party report of the Federation of Medical Royal Colleges.* London: Royal College of Physicians; 2000. 26pp.

4   Royal College of Physicians. *Acute medical care. The right person, in the right setting – first time.* Report of the Acute Medicine Task Force. London: Royal College of Physicians; Oct 2007. 76pp.

5   West Midlands Urgent Care Pathway Group. *Quality Standards for Acute Medical Units (AMUs).* West Bromwich, UK: West Midlands Quality Review Service and the Society for Acute Medicine; Jun 2012. 30pp. Available from: www.wmqi.westmidlands.nhs.uk/wmqrs/news/quality-standards-for-acute-medical-units-launched-today

6   Tian Y, Dixon A, Gao, H. *Emergency hospital admissions for ambulatory care sensitive conditions; identifying the potential for reductions.* Data Briefing. London: The King's Fund; 3 Apr 2012. 13pp. Available from: www.kingsfund.org.uk/publications/data-briefing-emergency-hospital-admissions-ambulatory-care-sensitive-conditions

7   Royal College of Physicians. *Acute care toolkit 4. Delivering a 12-hour, 7-day consultant presence on the acute medical unit.* London: RCP, 2012.

8   Royal College of Physicians. *Acute care toolkit 2: high quality acute care.* London: Royal College of Physicians; 2011.

9   Mort D, Lansdown M, Smith N, Protopapa K, Mason M. *For better, for worse? A review of the care of patients who died within 30 days of receiving systemic anti-cancer therapy.* London: National Confidential Enquiry into Patient Outcome and Death (NCEPOD); Nov 2008. 150pp.

05 High-Risk Patients Outside Intensive Care

Komal Ray, Jay Naik, Stuart Murdoch

Case History

A 48-year-old man with a recent diagnosis of non-seminomatous germ cell tumour, currently working full time as a company director and otherwise fit and well, is now undergoing chemotherapy. He presents 10 days after his second cycle of chemotherapy, with a three-day history of fatigue, feeling generally unwell, with pyrexia and a cough. He is sent for assessment.

What is the likely diagnosis?

What are the important components of initial management?

How can deteriorating patients be identified?

Background

What is the likely diagnosis? Is this patient high risk?

Sepsis is the likely diagnosis. It is a recognized and potentially fatal complication of anticancer treatment, particularly chemotherapy. Neutropenic sepsis (NS) is the second most common reason for hospital admission among children and young people with cancer, with approximately 4000 episodes occurring annually in the UK. Systemic therapies to treat cancer have a risk of reducing the bone marrow's ability to respond to infection by reducing its ability to produce neutrophils and alter the immune response.

Neutropenic sepsis is a medical emergency requiring immediate attention. These patients are very high risk as they can rapidly deteriorate and develop multiorgan failure and die. Patients receiving chemotherapy and radiotherapy should be warned about signs and symptoms of sepsis, which can occur during chemotherapy or up to six weeks after. Treatment and care should take into account patients' needs and preferences. Patients should be given verbal and written information on how and when to contact 24-hour specialist oncology advice, and how and when to seek emergency care (which may be at a site different from that where they receive their oncology treatment).

Time is of the essence in the management of these patients, and evidence suggests that outcomes worsen with delays in resuscitation and increased time to appropriate antibiotic treatment.

The mortality from sepsis if it is allowed to develop into severe sepsis is significant, and efforts have focused on early identification and treatment in an effort to limit progression.[1] Once identified, the goal of sepsis treatment is to eliminate the underlying infection by removal of infected tissue or implants alongside the use of antibiotics. The remainder of care is supportive, aimed at allowing the body to overcome the septic response and recover. As yet there is no established therapy which is used to treat sepsis – response to therapy is highly variable and a high mortality persists.

Screening tools have been introduced to identify patients at high risk of sepsis to ensure appropriate early treatment and management.[2] An example of this can be found in Figure 5.1. Each oncology department should have its own protocols for dealing with suspected NS.

Are any two of the following SIRS criteria present and new to the patient?

- Heart rate >90 beats/min
- Respiratory rate >20/min
- Abnormal temperature <36.0°C or >38.3°C
- Acutely altered mental state
- Blood glucose >7.7 mmol/l (in absence of diabetes)
- WCC <4/ >12 × 10⁹/l OR neutropenia (neutrophils <1 ×10⁹/l)

Think sepsis, consider source

- Chest (cough, sputum, pneumonia)
- Acute abdominal infection
- Meninigitis
- Urinary tract
- Wound infection
- Bloodstream – catheter related
- Other

Patient has SEPSIS

Look for organ dysfunction

- Systolic blood pressure <90mmHg or MAP <65mmHg
- Bilateral pulmonary infiltrates
- SpO₂ <90% unless O₂ given
- Platelet count <100,000
- Coagulopathy (INR >1.5 or APPT >60 seconds)
- Lactate >2 mmol/l
- Creatinine >177 mmol/l
- Bilirubin >34 mmol/l

If organ dysfunction present patient has severe sepsis

Figure 5.1 Sepsis screening tool. SIRS, systemic inflammatory response syndrome.

What are the important components of initial management?

Once sepsis has been identified it is important that initial care and treatment is given as soon as possible. The initial steps of management have been termed the 'Sepsis Six' pathway with an aim to complete within one hour.[3] The Sepsis Six consists of the following components, all of which should be delivered within the hour on suspicion of sepsis:

1. Deliver high-flow oxygen
2. Take blood cultures and other cultures, consider source control
3. Administer empirical intravenous (IV) antibiotics
4. Measure serum lactate or alternative
5. Start IV fluid resuscitation using Hartmann's or equivalent
6. Commence accurate urine output measurement.

Urinary catheterization should be considered early to allow accurate urine output measurement; however, it remains vital to monitor urine output even in the absence of catheterization. Local policies on antibiotics for urinary catheterization should be adhered to.

Evidence suggests that patients treated with this care bundle have better outcomes and spend less time in critical care than those patients who do not.

Oxygen

Oxygen for acutely hypoxic patients should aim to achieve a target saturation of 94%–98% (for those at risk of hypercapnic respiratory failure 88%–92% can be aimed for).[4] Initially oxygen should be given at a high concentration (15 litres per minute via a reservoir bag mask) and then reduced as appropriate.

Blood cultures and antibiotics

Appropriate antibiotics are a key principle in tackling sepsis, with evidence suggesting that delays in the administration of antibiotics are associated with increased risk of death.[5] The choice of antibiotics is difficult, but it should have a breadth of coverage to ensure adequate penetration and treatment of the likely source, very often using combinations of antibiotics. Ideally, specimens for culture and microscopy should be taken from all appropriate areas prior to antibiotic administration. Antibiotics should be reviewed regularly in light of microbiology results and in a bid to avoid toxicity and unwarranted use of broad-spectrum agents. National Institute for Health and Care Excellence (NICE) guidance suggests piperacillin/tazobactam as first-line therapy, with some scope for variation according to local antimicrobial resistance patterns.[6]

If appropriate, patients should receive physiotherapy to aid with the mobilization and expectoration of secretions. The use of culture specimens is ideal for guiding antibiotic treatment, and in some instances can help with the diagnosis of hard to detect organisms (*Pneumocystis* pneumonia for example). While the use of bronchoscopy is advocated to collect specimens, this may worsen a patient's condition and result in the need for ventilation when it could be avoided. The decision for bronchoscopy should be made in conjunction with an experienced respiratory physician and balanced against the risk of a patient's condition deteriorating.

Lactate measurement

This is a marker of organ perfusion; it is generally raised in patients who have inadequate perfusion of their tissues and resolves as resuscitation progresses and organ perfusion improves. The upper limit of normal for lactate is usually 1.6–2.0 mmol/l; it is higher in venous blood than arterial blood and the higher the level the greater the extent of hypoperfusion.

Fluid therapy and urine output

Fluids should be prescribed after a thorough assessment of a patient's volume status. Fluid challenges for hypotensive patients with previous cardiac problems should be 250–500 ml initially given as quickly as possible. Judging how often this should be repeated before considering the need for inotropes or pressure monitoring is difficult. The fluid challenge can be repeated if there is still improvement in blood pressure with each fluid challenge and if there is no evidence of fluid overload as judged by shortness of breath. It is very often necessary to give a patient several litres of fluid to resuscitate them. One approach is to raise the patient's legs and assess the blood pressure response to the increase in venous volume with this challenge; it can be reversed again by lowering the legs – this challenge is reported to represent a fluid bolus of approximately 500 ml.

Hartmann's solution is preferred as it is isotonic, but there is considerable debate about choice of fluid colloid vs crystalloid, etc. The most important aspect of fluid management is that a fluid is given as soon as possible to restore a patient's blood pressure.

Hypotension and hypovolaemia can lead to a decrease in urine output and potential kidney injury. The best way to avoid kidney injury is to ensure an adequate blood pressure and circulating volume. There is no place in this context for the use of diuretics or other agents in the avoidance of kidney injury. Hourly urine output measurement is useful in determining the adequacy of the blood pressure for the perfusion of the kidneys.

If the patient responds to treatment and is physiologically stable after resuscitation it may be appropriate for the patient to be nursed on the ordinary ward with an increased frequency of observations, avoiding the need for high dependency or intensive care.

Identification of the deteriorating patient

Early detection and initiation of treatment by appropriately skilled individuals is fundamental to achieving optimal outcomes for acutely unwell patients. To enable identification of deteriorating patients, considerable work has been done over the last ten years to introduce early warning scores which can be applied in any clinical area and used to determine the patient's risk of deteriorating. Recently, a national early warning score (NEWS) has been advocated for roll out across the country.[7] This score weights six physiological variables to alert individuals about a patient's condition. The proposed table (Table 5.1) weights abnormalities according to their deviation from normal, and the larger the score the higher the risk of the patient deteriorating (Table 5.2). The response to the abnormality will vary from institute to institute, but it is vital that individuals with appropriate knowledge and seniority are involved in looking after this group of patients. This service is often provided by critical care and outreach services which have developed to provide support to ward areas in looking after patients at risk of deterioration prior to critical care admission.

Table 5.1 National Early Warning Score (NEWS). Adapted from ref. 8.

Physiological parameters	3	2	1	0	1	2	3
Respiration rate	≤8		9-11	12-20		21-24	≥25
Oxygen saturations	≤91	92-93	94-95	≥96			
Any supplemental oxygen		YES		NO			
Temperature	≤35.0		35.1-36.0	36.1-38.0	38.1-39.0	≥39.1	
Systolic BP	≤90	91-100	101-110	111-219			≥220
Heart rate	≤40		41-50	51-90	91- 10	111-130	≥131
Level of consciousness				A			V, P, or U

The NEWS Score Initiative flowed from the Royal College of Physicians' NEWS Development and Implementation Group (NEWSDIG) report, and was jointly developed and funded in collaboration with: The Royal College of Physicians, The Royal College of Nursing, The National Outreach Forum, and NHS Training for Innovation

Table 5.2: **NEWS thresholds and triggers. As the clinical risk increases the seniority of the team responding and the time it takes for them to respond should increase. Different hospitals will have different team structures to respond.**

NEW Scores	Clinical risk
0	Low
Aggregate 1–4	
RED score* (Individual parameter scoring 3)	Medium
Aggregate 5–6	
Aggregate 7 or more	High

*RED score refers to an extreme variation in a single physiological parameter (i.e. a score of 3 on the NEWS chart, usually coloured red to aid identification and representing an extreme variation in a single physiological parameter). The consensus of the NEWSDIG was that extreme values in one physiological parameter (e.g. heart rate <40 beats per minute, or a respiratory rate of <8 per minute or a temperature of <35°C) could not be ignored and on its own required urgent clinical evaluation.

Further reading

1 Dellinger RP, Levy MM, Carlet JM, *et al.* Surviving Sepsis Campaign: International guidelines for management of severe sepsis and septic shock: 2008. *Crit Care Med* 2008; **36**: 296–327

2 Intensive Care Society. *Guidelines for the introduction of outreach services.* London: Intensive Care Society; 2002.

3   Survive Sepsis. [Internet] c.2012. Available from: http://survivesepsis.org

4   O'Driscoll BR, Howard LS, Davison AG; British Thoracic Society. BTS guideline for emergency oxygen use in adult patients. *Thorax* 2008; **63**(Suppl 6): vi1–vi68.

5   Kumar A, Roberts D, Wood KE, *et al.* Duration of hypotension before initiation of effective antimicrobial therapy is the critical determinant of survival in human septic shock. *Crit Care Med* 2006; **34**: 1589–96.

6   NICE [Internet]. *Neutropenic sepsis: prevention and management of neutropenic sepsis in cancer patients (CG151)*. London: National Institute for Health and Care Excellence; Sep 2012. Available from: http://guidance.nice.org.uk/CG151

7   Royal College of Physicians. *National Early Warning Score (NEWS): Standardising the assessment of acute-illness severity in the NHS*. Report of a working party. London: Royal College of Physicians; Jul 2012. 46pp.

8   NICE [Internet]. *Acutely ill patients in hospital: recognition of and response to acute illness in adults in hospital (CG50)*. London: National Institute for Health and Care Excellence; Jul 2007. Available from: www.nice.org.uk/cg50

PROBLEM

06 High-Dependency Unit Contribution

Komal Ray, Jay Naik, Stuart Murdoch

Case History

The patient discussed in Chapter 5 is now confirmed to have sepsis, and despite initial resuscitation and care on the ward has not improved. He is requiring increasing amounts of oxygen to maintain his saturations, has a high respiratory rate (>21 breaths/minute) and his breathing is laboured. His systolic blood pressure remains below 90 mmHg.

What should be done for this patient next?

Background

What should be done for this patient next?

This patient will have a score on an early warning system that will trigger review by senior medical staff and staff regularly involved in the care of critically ill patients.[1,2] Pending the introduction of a national early warning system,[3] many systems are currently used, all aimed at identifying acutely unwell patients and instituting prompt care. If a score is low but there is clinical concern about a patient it is appropriate that senior and skilled staff are involved at an early stage. Many young, previously fit patients are able to compensate and then deteriorate rapidly. It is invariably easier and more effective to deal with patients before they decompensate and organ dysfunction becomes established.

The severity of the illness at this point will require more intensive monitoring above the level of normal ward care. The frequency of observations of the patient should increase and standard physiological parameters should be monitored at least 12 hourly; as the patient becomes more unwell this frequency should increase appropriately. In a critical care unit the observations will usually be at least hourly and often continuously. As a patient's condition improves the frequency of observations should be reduced.

The team looking after the patient in consultation with the critical care team and the patient determine that the patient should be moved to a high-dependency unit (HDU).

The discussion will be the same as for any patient admitted to critical care – their desires and wishes and their potential for recovery, future life expectancy and underlying disease will play a part in this. High-dependency care is often referred to as 'Level 2 Care'; the levels of care come from the UK Department of Health document, *Comprehensive Critical Care*, and are outlined in Table 6.1.[4]

Level of care	Example
0	Need can be met on normal ward: • less frequent observation • Intravenous fluids
1	Ward care for the "sicker patient" • Oxygen therapy • Fluid boluses • More frequent observations • Established renal failure needing intermittent dialysis • Patients being monitored by critical care "outreach"
2	Patients requiring frequent observation • Patient receiving extended post-operative care • Receiving basic respiratory support • Single organ support • Patient stepped down from level 3 care • Usually one nurse to two patients
3	Patients receiving advanced respiratory support • Patients receiving two or more organ support • Usually one nurse to one patient

Table 6.1 **Levels of care**

Recent Developments

High-dependency care

On HDU, monitoring of basic physiological parameters should begin, usually assisted by an arterial line which allows continuous blood pressure measurement and regular arterial blood gases. This is in addition to continuous ECG monitoring, SpO_2 and urine output.

Respiratory support

The patient is hypoxic; to overcome this patients often increase their respiratory rate (one of the most sensitive indicators of critical illness). The initial way to treat hypoxia is to increase the percentage of inspired oxygen. In the first instance this should be 100% oxygen via a face-mask with an oxygen reservoir; oxygen can then be decreased to maintain a saturation of at least 94%.[5] Whilst there is concern about respiratory depression in patients with COPD, this should not prevent the administration of high concentratios of oxygen to hypoxic patients.

Oxygen is a drug and should be prescribed with clear guidance as to the monitoring needed and the objective of the oxygen. Those patients needing high percentages of oxygen in the long term will benefit from humidification of the gas to prevent drying of secretions and heat loss (from cold gas). This can be done by the use of humidifiers and Hi-Flow oxygen.

If the patient's saturations (SpO$_2$) are not maintained with supplemental oxygen, consideration can be given to non-invasive methods of respiratory support – this avoids the need for intubation and the use of sedative drugs. The most basic method is application of continuous positive airway pressure (CPAP) with the delivery of a continuous flow of inspired gas against a fixed pressure. One method by which CPAP may work is by reducing airway collapse and improving oxygenation, but this does not generally result in increased carbon dioxide clearance. While there is still controversy about the use of CPAP and other methods of non-invasive ventilation for acute respiratory failure, it is believed that the more widespread use of such techniques has reduced the risk of complications from invasive ventilation and improved outcomes for patients.[6] However it is vital that such techniques are used in a suitable critical care environment with staff able to quickly respond to deteriorations in a patient's condition and institute invasive ventilation if needed.

Cardiovascular support

Hypotension results in poor perfusion of the major organ systems, resulting in organ dysfunction (manifest by cold, blue periphery; reduced renal output; and altered conscious levels). Other markers of hypoperfusion include blood lactate, which is raised in shock states, and a metabolic acidosis indicating poor organ perfusion and hypoxic tissues. Initial management should ensure the patient is adequately filled. On HDU it is possible to continuously measure the patient's blood pressure and their central venous pressure (CVP).

The aim of fluid resuscitation should be to ensure that the patient perfuses their organs appropriately. Central venous pressure, whilst not without drawbacks, can be used to guide appropriate fluid therapy with fluid given until the CVP is above a nominal figure (typically 10-15 mmHg). However, fluid resuscitation is often inadequate to completely restore blood pressure. Sepsis can cause vasodilatation, which can be treated by the use of vasoconstrictors. These drugs must be given by means of a central line, and act on peripheral vessels to cause them to constrict and increase the blood pressure.

Renal support

Once the patient has been adequately filled and an adequate mean arterial pressure obtained there is little further that can be done to reduce acute kidney injury (AKI). Avoidance of nephrotoxic drugs (or alteration of their dose) and appropriate use of radiocontrast dyes for imaging can all help to reduce the risk of AKI in acutely unwell patients. However, only adequate hydration has been proven to reduce the incidence of AKI in this group of patients.

Other organ systems

It is important in any critically ill patient that attention is paid to all organ systems. Apropos of this, the 'Surviving Sepsis' campaign has put together a list of interventions that should be addressed for all patients; this includes DVT prophylaxis, stress ulcer prophylaxis, glucose control and renal replacement therapy, amongst others.[3] One of the key elements of this is the need to ensure adequate nutrition – this helps reduce the starvation response, and may result in less muscle loss.

Future planning

Whilst the patient is in the HDU, it is important to consider what the patient would want in the event of their deterioration.[8] This will allow decisions to be made when a patient may no longer be able to communicate those decisions for themselves, and may help them and their family appreciate the seriousness of their condition. Severe sepsis has a high mortality rate even with optimal medical treatment, and it is important that both patients and families recognize this and are prepared for it. This discussion should involve both the critical care team, who have knowledge and experience of the outcomes of sepsis in critically ill patients, and the oncology team, who will know the patient and their prognosis from the underlying disease.

Further reading

1   NICE [Internet]. *Acutely ill patients in hospital: recognition of and response to acute illness in adults in hospital (CG50)*. London: National Institute for Health and Care Excellence; Jul 2007. Available from: www.nice.org.uk/cg50

2   Royal College of Physicians. *Acute medical care. The right person, in the right setting – first time.* Report of the Acute Medicine Task Force. London: Royal College of Physicians; Oct 2007. 76pp.

3   Royal College of Physicians. *National Early Warning Score (NEWS): Standardising the assessment of acute-illness severity in the NHS.* Report of a working party. London: Royal College of Physicians; Jul 2012. 46pp.

4   Department of Health. *Comprehensive critical care: a review of adult critical care services.* London: Department of Health; 25 May 2000. 32pp.

5   O'Driscoll BR, Howard LS, Davison AG; British Thoracic Society. BTS guideline for emergency oxygen use in adult patients. *Thorax* 2008; **63**(Suppl 6): vi1–vi68.

6   Bello G, De Pascale G, Antonelli M. Noninvasive ventilation for the immunocompromised patient: always appropriate? *Curr Opin Crit Care* 2012; **18**: 54–60.

7   Survive Sepsis. [Internet] c.2012. Available from: http://survivesepsis.org

8   Dying Matters Coalition, National End of Life Care Programme, University of Nottingham. *Planning for your future care: A guide.* Published by the National End of Life Care Programme; 1 Feb 2012. 16pp.

07 Intensive Care Unit for Cancer Patients

Komal Ray, Jay Naik, Stuart Murdoch

Case History

The patient discussed in Chapters 5 and 6 has been in the high-dependency unit (HDU); despite initial improvements in his condition he is now deteriorating. He is hypoxic and is being given continuous positive airway pressure (CPAP) therapy for respiratory failure, requiring 90% oxygen to achieve Po_2 8 kPa and looks increasingly tired. Despite adequate fluids, the patient is hypotensive and has been anuric for the last eight hours.

How should this patient's condition be managed in an intensive care setting?

Background

The patient is reaching the limit of what the HDU can offer. If the patient's care is to continue with an aim of achieving recovery he will need support for his respiratory system – most likely in the form of positive pressure ventilation. He will need inotropes to support his hypotension, and will need renal support in the form of dialysis or haemofiltration. While some of these therapies can be provided in an HDU setting, the need for these therapies together will necessitate admission to an intensive care unit (ICU).

How should this patient's condition be managed in an intensive care setting?

The provision of ventilation is often via an endotracheal tube, which necessitates the administration of sedatives so that the patient can tolerate the tube. This initially renders the patient unconscious. A side effect of many sedatives is a drop in blood pressure, which may need further treatment. The endotracheal tube can later be removed as the patient's condition improves and they are able to breathe independently, or may be replaced by a tracheostomy which is more easily tolerated by patients and is believed to allow easier weaning of the patient. The use of an endotracheal tube increases the risk of the patient developing a nosocomial pneumonia. Steps are taken to reduce this risk, including the use of antiseptic mouthwash and good oral hygiene.

Hypotension is treated by ensuring adequate fluid resuscitation of the patient, guided by central venous pressure (CVP) or other measures of filling. Then the provision of inotropes and vasoconstrictors can be used to improve the blood pressure. The most commonly used drug is noradrenaline (norepinephrine), which acts to improve vascular tone and blood pressure; in patients with inadequate cardiac output dobutamine or adrenaline (epinephrine) can be used to improve cardiac function.

Many patients in the ICU will suffer an acute kidney injury (AKI).[1] This is defined as any of the following:

- Serum creatinine rises by 26 mol/l within 48 hours
- Serum creatinine rises 1.5-fold from the reference value, which is known or presumed to have occurred within one week
- Urine output is <0.5 ml/kg/h for more than six consecutive hours.

To prevent AKI the patient should be adequately resuscitated and blood pressure maintained at a level which will ensure renal perfusion. There is no evidence that diuretics or dopamine will alter the course of renal injury, but it is important that nephrotoxic drugs are avoided – NSAIDs, ACE inhibitors and aminoglycosides. Whilst contrast media are toxic, a ris-benefit analysis must be made when considering the need for radiological investigation and the risk this poses to the kidneys.

To compensate for AKI it is possible to consider renal haemodialysis/filtration, usually offered via a central line which can cope with the flow needed to filter blood. Patients may have to be anticoagulated for this treatment using heparin, which may present a bleeding risk. Renal support can be offered acutely for acute disturbances of potassium or pH, or in instances of fluid overload. Rises in urea and creatinine do not usually necessitate acute filtration.

The ICU will also be delivering high-quality basic care, such as nutrition, glycaemic control, central line management and appropriate antibiotics, with the aim of ensuring no further deterioration in a patient's condition. There is currently no definitive treatment for sepsis despite years of investigation and several false dawns.

Dilemmas in critical care

One of the most difficult questions relating to critical care is determining when the patient should continue to be offered support or whether treatment has become futile. Regardless of an oncology diagnosis, the mortality from severe sepsis is high, a recent study in Europe suggesting a mortality as high as 40%.[2] Mortality increases with advanced age, number of organs failing and comorbidities. This information should be borne in mind in any discussion with the patient and family irrespective of a cancer diagnosis. For some patients with a guarded prognosis due to underlying disease, consideration must be given to the purpose and utility of critical care.

Early experience of critically ill patients with cancer demonstrated poor outcomes and few survivors. To an extent this became a self-fulfilling prophecy, with patients either not being referred, or those that were referred often being severely unwell with little chance of recovery. In the 1980s mortality rates as high as 80% in ICU were reported in haematology patients;[3] a comment in a paper reporting UK experience demonstrated similar poor outcomes with few surviving to be discharged from hospital.[4]

A recent review of the UK critical care experience involving patients admitted to ICU with an underlying haematological malignancy demonstrated an ICU mortality of over 40% and a hospital mortality of nearly 60%.[5] While a single UK centre review demonstrated better short-term outcomes in critical care (30% mortality), six-month mortality approached 80% (Figure 7.1).[6]

It is against this background of poor outcomes that critical care decisions relating to admission and continuation of care are made. The best method of improving patient outcome is early detection and treatment of sepsis on the ward prior to coming to a critical care environment.

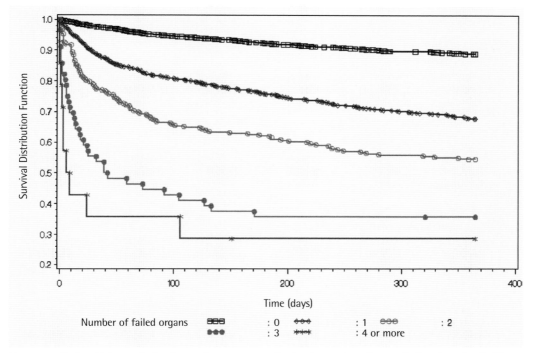

Figure 7.1 Kaplan–Meier survival estimates for 1-year mortality by the number of organ dysfunctions. Survival in days according to the number of dysfunctional organs is shown out to 1 year. (Adapted from ref. 7 with permission.)

Conclusion

The preceding case study (Chapters 5, 6 and 7) detail the specific steps to follow for patients being treated for sepsis. The emphasis for oncology patients, therefore, should be on early detection and intervention to prevent and treat clinical deterioration. This should include pathways to rapid identification of the deteriorating patient, early intervention for organ dysfunction, and the administration of broad-spectrum antibiotics to cover likely infective agents.

It is key that all staff involved in the care of patients at risk of deterioration are familiar with the identification and initial treatment of this group of patients. The early involvement of critical care (outreach) teams will support the parent team looking after a patient, and may allow intervention on the ward to prevent further deterioration and facilitate escalation of care as appropriate.

For those patients requiring extra input, the HDU can offer more intensive monitoring and generally single organ support, whilst the ICU can offer multiorgan support including endotracheal intubation and haemofiltration. However, it is worth keeping in mind that mortality escalates sharply with an increasing number of failing organs.

In all settings a careful assessment of the context of the patient's illness and wishes, including clear escalation decisions, prior to committing to higher levels of intervention will ensure the most appropriate care for the patient.

After careful discussion and consideration by the clinical teams, the patient described above was accepted onto the ICU and received full active treatment including ventilation, cardiac support and renal dialysis. Despite this effort, after three days it was apparent that the patient was not responding to treatment and was continuing to deteriorate. After discussion with the family it was agreed that the emphasis of care should switch to symptom control. It is impossible to know if earlier treatment of the infection would have altered his clinical outcome; however, the limited available evidence does suggest that early identification and appropriate treatment of infection in the general clinical population may improve outcomes.

Further reading

1 Lewington A, Kanagasundaram S. *Acute Kidney Injury, 5th edition.* Clinical Practice Guidelines. Petersfield, Hants.: The Renal Association (UK); 8 Mar 2011. Available from: www.renal.org/Clinical/GuidelinesSection/Guidelines.aspx

2 Levy MM, Artigas A, Phillips GS, *et al.* Outcomes of the Surviving Sepsis Campaign in intensive care units in the USA and Europe: a prospective cohort study. *Lancet Infect Dis* 2012; **12**: 919–24.

3 Peters S, Meadows A, Gracey D. Outcome of respiratory failure in hematologic malignancy. *Chest* 1988; **94**: 99–102.

4 Yau E, Rohatiner AZ, Lister TA, Hinds CJ. Long term prognosis and quality of life following intensive care for life-threatening complications of haematological malignancy. *Br J Cancer* 1991; **64**(5): 938–42

5 Hampshire PA, Welch CA, McCrossan LA, Francis K, Harrison DA. Admission factors associated with hospital mortality in patients with haematological malignancy admitted to UK adult, general critical care units: a secondary analysis of the ICNARC Case Mix Programme Database. *Crit Care* 2009; **13**: R137.

6 McGrath S, Chatterjee F, Whiteley C, Ostermann M. ICU and 6-month outcome of oncology patients in the intensive care unit. *QJM* 2010; **103**: 397–403.

7 Shapiro N, Howell MD, Bates DW, Angus DC, Ngo L, Talmor D. The association of sepsis syndrome and organ dysfunction with mortality in emergency department patients with suspected infection. *Ann Emerg Med* 2006; **48**: 583–90, 590.e1.

PROBLEM

08 Managing Acute Issues in Oncology in Canada and the United States

Monika K. Krzyzanowska, Jennifer L. Malin

Cancer is a leading cause of morbidity and mortality in North America. In 2012, approximately 186 400 new cases of cancer and 75 700 cancer deaths were expected in Canada,[1] and 1 638 910 new cases of cancer and 577 190 cancer deaths were expected in the United States.[2] Despite significant differences in the organization and funding of healthcare delivery in the two countries, concerns regarding quality of care exist around issues such as access and medication errors in medicine in general,[3–5] and in cancer specifically,[6,7] coupled with rapidly escalating healthcare costs.[8–10] These concerns have led to substantial interest over the last decade in reforming healthcare delivery at the policy as well as the clinic level in both countries, with significant changes expected in the near future.

There are significant differences in how cancer services are delivered and paid for in the two countries. In Canada, most health services, including cancer care, are paid for publicly with legal residents of Canada being entitled to receive medically necessary services without co-payment. Each of Canada's ten provinces and three territories is responsible for the organization of health services delivered within their jurisdiction. When it comes to cancer care specifically, most Canadian provinces have elected to develop provincial agencies such as Cancer Care Ontario[11] or the British Columbia Cancer Agency[12] to organize and deliver cancer services. As a result, most Canadian provinces have a centralized approach to cancer services delivery, with networks of regional cancer centres and various affiliated institutions providing the vast majority of specialized services such as radiation and chemotherapy. In the USA, by contrast, a number of systems exist for paying for health services, including cancer care. These are composed of public programmes, such as Medicare (for individuals older than 65), Medicaid (for low-income families and individuals) and the Veterans Affairs Health Care System (for veterans), in addition to a wide variety of private insurance plans usually obtained as part of an employment package. There is also a substantial proportion of Americans younger than 65 who are uninsured; however, with the passage of the Patient Protection and Affordable Care Act in 2010, most Americans are expected to have access to health insurance either through publicly funded programmes, employer-sponsored plans, or by purchasing individual coverage through health insurance exchanges. Given the heterogeneous financing of healthcare in the US, most cancer care is delivered through a fee for service model, with the majority of cancer patients receiving care in community-based settings by private practitioners. Whilst this may provide patients with many providers to choose from, it can also result in care that is delivered across multiple settings and is often fragmented.

One of the biggest challenges facing cancer care delivery in both Canada and the US is the management of acute problems, such as treatment of adverse events, or complications relating to the cancer itself, especially in patients with advanced disease.

Population-based studies suggest that cancer patients across the continuum of care, from diagnosis through to end-of-life, frequently experience problems that require them to seek attention in an acute care setting. A Canadian study found that 76 759 out of 91 561 patients (84%) who died of cancer in Ontario between 2002 and 2005 made 194 017 visits to the emergency department (ED) in the last six months of life, and that 40% of these visits were made in the last two weeks of life.[13] In a 2008 study of ED visits in the state of North Carolina, 37 760 of 4 190 911 ED visits that year (0.9%) were made by 27 644 cancer patients.[14] The three most common reasons for ED visits were pain, respiratory distress and gastrointestinal complaints. Frequent ED visits and hospitalizations have also been described in patients receiving chemotherapy for early stage breast cancer.[15,16]

The high number of emergency room visits and hospitalizations among cancer patients suggests that novel models of care delivery for acute issues in oncology are sorely needed in North America. At present, management of acute issues in oncology has focused on three aspects of care: use of preventative strategies, patient education and telephone support. Guidelines have been developed recommending appropriate antiemetics for prevention of chemotherapy and radiotherapy-induced nausea and vomiting,[17] and prophylaxis for febrile neutropenia.[18] All patients undergo some level of patient education informally by the physician and/or nurse in the oncology clinic. Some centres have also developed formal chemotherapy teaching classes that provide patients and their caregivers with information regarding potential side effects and their management. However, less is known about the effectiveness of patient education with respect to their ability to self-manage side effects and this is an area of active research. In addition, most centres provide access to telephone advice for urgent care issues although fewer centres have the capacity to see patients in urgent care clinics or can provide advice outside of clinic hours. Furthermore, present telephone support tends to be reactive rather than proactive. For specific acute issues, such as febrile neutropenia, protocols for management of low-risk patients in the outpatient setting have been developed, although their rate of uptake is unknown.[19]

To deal with the frequent unmet acute needs of cancer patients and the fragmented nature of care a number of novel models are currently being explored in North America. In the US, the concept of the 'oncology medical home' has been gaining momentum. The idea behind the oncology medical home arose from the patient-centred medical home programme created on the basis of National Committee for Quality Assurance (NCQA) standards.[20] The key components of this model are greater responsibility by the oncology team for disease management and care coordination, and more active patient engagement. The goals of the programme are to improve quality of care and patient satisfaction while optimizing care efficiency. This is felt to lead to cost savings, with preliminary evaluations in the primary care setting showing encouraging results.[21,22] Several oncology groups around the US are currently adopting the oncology medical home concept and their experiences with the model are expected soon.[23]

Another major issue in oncology in North America is management of patients with advanced cancers near the end of life. Studies have found that a significant proportion of patients with end-stage cancer receive aggressive care at the end of life, defined as chemotherapy close to death, admissions to hospital and intensive care units within the last few weeks of life, and underuse of hospice services.[24,25] Whilst the rates of aggressive care have generally been higher in the US than Canada,[25] both countries have identified end of life care as an important target for quality improvement. This is further reinforced by recent studies, which have shown significant benefits of early palliative care and better end-of-life care on survival,[26] quality of life[27] and aggressiveness of care in patients with end-stage cancer.[28,29] There are significant efforts in both countries to improve quality of end-of-life care that focus on systematic and comprehensive symptom management[30] and integration of palliative care early and in a comprehensive fashion.[31]

One of the main approaches to improving quality of cancer care in Canada and the US has been through the use of quality measurement to drive change. In Ontario, Canada's largest province, public reporting of quality of the cancer system through its Cancer System Quality Index has been in place since 2005.[32] Gaps in care identified through this index have been used to drive quality improvement in the province, especially in access to services. More recently, the Canadian Partnership Against Cancer, has undertaken pan-Canadian tracking of cancer quality that is reported in an annual report.[33] In the US, a number of cancer organizations have developed formal quality measurement systems, including the American Society of Clinical Oncology's Quality of Oncology Practice Initiative (QOPI)[34,35], the American College of Surgeons' Commission on Cancer Rapid Quality Reporting System,[36] and the Center for Medicare and Medicaid Services Physician Quality Reporting Initiative (PQRI) also includes quality measures relevant to oncology.[37] The QOPI is a practice-based quality measurement initiative that was initially developed by a group of community oncologists as a tool to evaluate adherence with processes of care. The programme continues to grow and evolve, and is currently being used by approximately 10% of American oncology practices.[38] Until recently, the majority of these quality reporting programmes have been voluntary, but with the establishment of accountable care organizations as part of the 2010 Affordable Care Act all American physicians participating in Medicare, including those providing cancer services, will be required to participate in the PQRI effective 2013 or face financial penalties.[39]

Current models of cancer care in Canada and the US are expensive and often inadequate to respond to the acute needs of cancer patients across the continuum of care. Novel multifaceted models that promote patient engagement and a comprehensive approach to care are currently being developed and may change the way acute problems are managed in cancer patients in North America in the near future. Quality measurement has and continues to be a widely used tool in both countries to drive transformation of health care delivery to improve quality of care and foster fiscal sustainability.

Further reading

1   Canadian Cancer Society's Steering Committee on Cancer Statistics. *Canadian Cancer Statistics 2012*. Toronto, ON: Canadian Cancer Society; May 2012. Available from: www.cancer.ca/statistics

2   American Cancer Society. *Cancer Facts & Figures 2012*. Atlanta, Ga.: American Cancer Society; 2012.

3   Institute of Medicine. *Crossing the Quality Chasm: A New Health System for the 21st Century*. Washington, D.C.: National Academy Press; 1 Mar 2001. 359pp.

4   Institute of Medicine. *To Err Is Human: Building a Safer Health System*. Washington, D.C.: National Academy Press; 1 Nov 1999. 311pp.

5   Baker GR, Norton PG, Flintoft V, *et al.* The Canadian Adverse Events Study: the incidence of adverse events among hospital patients in Canada. *CMAJ* 2004; **170**(11): 1678–86.

6   Cancer Quality Council of Ontario. *Strengthening the Quality of Cancer Services in Ontario.* Toronto, ON: Cancer Care Ontario; 2003.

7   Simone JV, Hewitt M, eds. *Ensuring Quality Cancer Care.* Washington, D.C.: National Academy Press; 1999.

8   Meropol NJ, Schrag D, Smith TJ, *et al.* American Society of Clinical Oncology guidance statement: the cost of cancer care. *J Clin Oncol* 2009; **27**(23): 3868–74.

9   Young RA, DeVoe JE. Who will have health insurance in the future? An updated projection. *Ann Fam Med* 2012; **10**(2): 156–62.

10   Elkin EB, Bach PB. Cancer's next frontier: addressing high and increasing costs. *JAMA* 2010; **303**(11): 1086–7.

11   Cancer Care Ontario [Internet]. Toronto, ON: Cancer Care Ontario; c.2009–13. Available from: www.cancercare.on.ca

12   British Columbia Cancer Agency [Internet]. Vancouver, BC: BC Cancer Agency; c.2013. Available from: www.bccancer.bc.ca

13   Barbera L, Taylor C, Dudgeon D. Why do patients with cancer visit the emergency department near the end of life? *CMAJ* 2010; **182**(6): 563–8.

14   Mayer DK, Travers D, Wyss A, Leak A, Waller A. Why do patients with cancer visit emergency departments? Results of a 2008 population study in North Carolina. *J Clin Oncol* 2011; **29**(19): 2683–8.

15   Hassett MJ, O'Malley AJ, Pakes JR, Newhouse JP, Earle CC. Frequency and cost of chemotherapy-related serious adverse effects in a population sample of women with breast cancer. *J Natl Cancer Inst* 2006; **98**(16): 1108–17.

16   Enright K, Grunfeld E, Yun L, *et al.* Acute care utilization among women receiving adjuvant chemotherapy for early breast cancer. *J Clin Oncol* 2012; **30**(Suppl 27): Abstr 65.

17   Basch E, Prestrud AA, Hesketh PJ, *et al.* Antiemetics: American Society of Clinical Oncology clinical practice guideline update. *J Clin Oncol* 2011; **29**(31): 4189–98.

18   Smith TJ, Khatcheressian J, Lyman GH, *et al.* 2006 update of recommendations for the use of white blood cell growth factors: an evidence-based clinical practice guideline. *J Clin Oncol* 2006; **24**(19): 3187–205.

19   Freifeld AG, Sepkowitz KA. No place like home? Outpatient management of patients with febrile neutropenia and low risk. *J Clin Oncol* 2011; **29**(30): 3952–4.

20   Sprandio JD. Oncology patient-centered medical home. *J Oncol Pract* 2012; **8**(3 Suppl): 47s–49s.

21   Harbrecht MG, Latts LM. Colorado's Patient-Centered Medical Home Pilot met numerous obstacles, yet saw results such as reduced hospital admissions. *Health Aff (Millwood)* 2012; **31**(9): 2010-7.

22   Raskas RS, Latts LM, Hummel JR, Wenners D, Levine H, Nussbaum SR. Early results show WellPoint's patient-centered medical home pilots have met some goals for costs, utilization, and quality. *Health Aff (Millwood)* 2012; **31**(9): 2002-9.

23   Bosserman LD, Verrilli D, McNatt W. Partnering with a payer to develop a value-based medical home pilot: a West Coast practice's experience. *J Oncol Pract* 2012; **8**(3 Suppl): 38s–40s.

24 Earle CC, Neville BA, Landrum MB, Ayanian JZ, Block SD, Weeks JC. Trends in the aggressiveness of cancer care near the end of life. *J Clin Oncol* 2004; **22**(2): 315–21.

25 Ho TH, Barbera L, Saskin R, Lu H, Neville BA, Earle CC. Trends in the aggressiveness of end-of-life cancer care in the universal health care system of Ontario, Canada. *J Clin Oncol* 2011; **29**(12): 1587–91.

26 Temel JS, Greer JA, Muzikansky A,, *et al*. Early palliative care for patients with metastatic non-small-cell lung cancer. *N Engl J Med* 2010; **363**(8): 733–42.

27 Zimmermann C, Swami N, Rodin G, *et al*. Cluster-randomized trial of early palliative care for patients with metastatic cancer. *J Clin Oncol* 2012; **30**(Suppl): Abstr 9003.

28 Wright AA, Zhang B, Ray A, *et al*. Associations between end-of-life discussions, patient mental health, medical care near death, and caregiver bereavement adjustment. *JAMA* 2008; **300**(14): 1665–73.

29 Mack JW, Cronin A, Keating NL, *et al*. Associations between end-of-life discussion characteristics and care received near death: a prospective cohort study. *J Clin Oncol* 2012; **30**(35): 4387–95.

30 Gilbert JE, Howell D, King S, *et al*. Quality improvement in cancer symptom assessment and control: the Provincial Palliative Care Integration Project (PPCIP). *J Pain Symptom Manage* 2012; **43**(4): 663–78.

31 Smith TJ, Temin S, Alesi ER, *et al*. American Society of Clinical Oncology provisional clinical opinion: the integration of palliative care into standard oncology care. *J Clin Oncol* 2012; **30**(8): 880–7.

32 Cancer System Quality Index (CSQI) 2013. [Internet]. Toronto, ON: Cancer Quality Council of Ontario; c.2013. [Accessed 18 Dec 2012] Available from: www.csqi.on.ca

33 Canadian Partnership Against Cancer. *The 2012 Cancer System Performance Report*. Toronto, ON: Canadian Partnership Against Cancer; Dec 2012. 196pp.

34 Neuss MN, Desch CE, McNiff KK, *et al*. A process for measuring the quality of cancer care: the Quality Oncology Practice Initiative. *J Clin Oncol* 2005; **23**(25): 6233–9.

35 Jacobson JO, Neuss MN, McNiff KK, *et al*. Improvement in oncology practice performance through voluntary participation in the Quality Oncology Practice Initiative. *J Clin Oncol* 2008; **26**(11): 1893–8.

36 Stewart AK, McNamara E, Gay EG, Banasiak J, Winchester DP. The Rapid Quality Reporting System—a new quality of care tool for CoC-accredited cancer programs. *J Registry Manag* 2011; **38**(1): 61–3.

37 Federman AD, Keyhani S. Physicians' participation in the Physicians' Quality Reporting Initiative and their perceptions of its impact on quality of care. *Health Policy* 2011; **102**(2–3): 229–34.

38 Jacobson JO. Quality oncology practice initiative turns seven. *J Oncol Pract* 2009; **5**(6): 268.

39 VanLare JM, Blum JD, Conway PH. Linking performance with payment: implementing the Physician Value-Based Payment Modifier. *JAMA* 2012; **308**(20): 2089–90.

09 Managing Acute Issues in Oncology in Australasia

Bridget Robinson

The biggest challenges to offering acute cancer services in Australasia come from the widely dispersed populations in the two countries, a burgeoning demand for oncology care due to an increasing population (especially the elderly), and an increase in more effective but complex therapies. The population distribution of Australia and New Zealand is shown in Tables 9.1 and 9.2. Australia has 22.3 million people spread over 7.66 million km² (approx. 3/km²); although 64% live in capital cities of each state, the remainder are widely spread, mainly near the coast. New South Wales (NSW) and Victoria have 57.3% of the Australian population, but just 13.4% of the land area, whilst Northern Territory has 1% of the population (of whom 30% are indigenous) on 17.5% of the land area.[1-3] New Zealand has 4.2 million people, 46% in the eight largest cities, spread over 0.27 million km² (approx. 15/km²), which is similar in area to Great Britain (where there are approx. 260 people per km²).[4]

Table 9.1 Australia population distribution, by state or territory

	Population, millions *	% of total population	% land area[†]	Indigenous % peoples[¶]	Population in capital city, %
New South Wales	7.23	32.4	10.4	2.3	63
Victoria	5.55	24.9	3.0	0.7	73
Queensland	4.51	20.2	22.5	3.6	67
Western Australia	2.29	10.3	33.0	3.4	74
South Australia	1.64	7.3	12.7	1.9	73
Tasmania	0.51	2.3	0.9	4.0	43
Northern Territory	0.23	1.0	17.5	30.7	34
ACT	0.36	1.6	<1	1.3	98
All Australia	22.33	100.0	100	2.6	64

* Australian Bureau of Statistics, at 30 June 2010. www.abs.gov.au (1)
¶ Australian Bureau of Statistics, www.abs.gov.au (2)
†total land area 7 659 861 km², Geoscience Australia, www.ga.gov.au (3)
  ACT Australian Capital Territory

Table 9.2 Population distribution in New Zealand (NZ), by cancer network region

Cancer network	No. DHBs	No. cancer centres	Population (M)	Population % NZ	Population Maori %	Population % Pacifica %	Rurality of DHBs: mean or range
Northern	4	1	1.54	37	13.5	11.9	0.2%–49%
Midland	3	1	0.63	16	23	3	20%
Central	8	2	1.00	24	17	4	1%–27%
Southern	5	2	1.00	24	8	1.6	13%–42%
All NZ	21	6	4.2	100	14.9	6	14%

DHB District Health Board
Statistics from New Zealand 2006 census, cited in (4)
www.northerncancernetwork.org.nz/ (5)
www.midlandcancernetwork.org.nz/ (6)
www.centralcancernetwork.org.nz/ (7)
www.southerncancernetwork.org.nz/ (8)

The cancer incidence in 2008 was 112 304 (with 39 884 deaths) in Australia,[9] and 20 317 (8566 deaths) in New Zealand.[10] A simple assessment shows that cancer mortality was 35.5% and 42%, respectively. There were 168 linear particle accelerators (known as linacs) in Australia in 2011, including 60 (36%) in private centres, with a range of population of 92 000 per linac in ACT and 182 000 in Western Australia, and two linacs covering the Northern Territory.[11] New Zealand is served by 29 linacs, five (19%) in private cancer centres.[12] In Australasia, chemotherapy is usually prescribed by medical oncologists: in Australia these number one per 78 000 population, with an average case load of 270 first assessments per year.[13,14] In New Zealand there is one per 101 000 population, with an average case load of 177 first assessments per year.[15] Radiation oncology case load averages 250–275 first assessments per year.[16]

Both countries have demonstrated inequities of outcome, due in part to the dispersed rural and remote populations, and these are especially associated with indigenous peoples, including New Zealand Maori and Pacific peoples.[4,17–20] These inequities come from barriers to prompt referral with a suspected new cancer diagnosis. This reduces access to adjuvant therapy. They have problems also in relation to access to specialist units, access to acute care for therapy complications and access to palliative care. In 2006, the Clinical Oncology Society of Australia (COSA) mapped cancer services in regional and rural Australia, identifying 161 regional hospitals which administered chemotherapy, with a 98% response rate to the questionnaire. Only 21% had a resident medical oncologist, 7% a radiation oncology unit, 6% a surgical oncologist, 24% a palliative care specialist, and 39% a dedicated oncology counselling service. In only 61% of these hospitals was chemotherapy given by chemotherapy-trained nurses. This situation has prompted national cancer control initiatives in Australia, followed by New Zealand, both of which have adopted features of cancer managed care networks developed in the UK.

The Cancer Council of Australia, together with COSA and the National Cancer Control Initiative, made 12 recommendations in a 2003 report entitled *Optimising*

Cancer Care in Australia.[22] These recommendations included: integrated multidisciplinary care; improved cancer journey, palliative care and access to clinical trials; better psycho-oncology; improvements in radiation therapy and access to pharmaceuticals; and travel support and bridging gaps for special populations. A national 'Task Force on Cancer' was recommended to implement the reforms. The Cancer Australia Act 2006 provided for national leadership for cancer control, and the establishment of Cancer Australia.[23] Implementation is occurring at state level, starting with the 'Cancer Services Framework for Victoria' in 2003, which created integrated cancer services in metropolitan Melbourne and rural/regional integrated centres with five levels of service.[24] This was followed by the 'NSW Cancer Plan' in 2004.[19,25]

In New Zealand a task force produced 'The New Zealand Cancer Control Strategy Action Plan 2005-2010', leading to establishment of the Cancer Control Council in 2005 (Cancer Control NZ since 2010)[26] and four regional cancer networks in 2006, which were charged with reducing inequalities as well as waiting times. Six cancer centres were identified and each of these has clinician-initiated multidisciplinary meetings, provides chemotherapy and radiation, manages acute problems, and is linked to several peripheral centres where chemotherapy is administered. Some of the peripheral centres have resident specialist medical oncologists and others visiting medical and/or radiation oncologists. Acute problems and complications affecting peripheral patients are managed by their general practitioner or at their local hospital. Care pathways for neutropenic sepsis and acute referrals with new problems are focused around specialist nurses who facilitate patient review, although there is a considerable variation in the support for patients in the community both in cities and rural areas.

In Australia, acute care of cancer patients in remote areas has been supported by extra training for nurses and non-specialist doctors, e.g. through educational workshops about chemotherapy[27] and an online programme for palliative care.[28] Clinicians use treatment and chemotherapy guidelines, 'tumour stream' guidelines, and national information resources such as the 'eviQ' portal developed by the Cancer Institute of NSW.[29] Telehealth is increasingly used for patient assessment, multidisciplinary discussions and education[30]. Whilst CT scans are undertaken in the treatment location in remote centres, the patients are assessed remotely in the regional centre by the appropriate radiation oncologist to speed up radiotherapy planning.[19,30,31] Each Australian state has a cancer network, 'canNET', which, like the New Zealand networks, links all the contributors to cancer care with common guidelines and more streamlined care.[19] Despite progress, deficiencies in Australian rural oncology services persist, including travel support and shortage of visiting oncologist time. It has been proposed that regional rather than metropolitan centres offer outreach services which would be closer and more frequent.[31] Cancer survival in rural and remote areas in Australia still lags metropolitan centres, including for common cancers such as breast and colon.[32]

The predicted increase in cancer patient numbers by 40% between 2007 and 2020 in Australia,[33] and doubling of the medical oncology workload in New Zealand over 15 years is expected to outstrip available medical oncologists.[13,14,34] This has prompted initiatives to increase specialist nurses and give additional training to general practitioners in the main centres as well as regionally. New Zealand has drawn from Australian experience, meaning increased capacity will be generated by funding improved service configurations and workforce models, with cancer coordinators to fast-track the patient journey, better resourced multidisciplinary meetings, and national tumour standards for the main cancer types.[34] There is a national approach to information technology support, exemplified by a South Island Clinical Cancer Information System.[35] The plan has also drawn from the Australian system in categorizing levels of oncology services. It has been suggested that radiation oncologists might be dual-trained to meet the increasing chemotherapy demands.[36]

Palliative care is nationally supported in both countries, with national standards in Australia[37] and a Palliative Care Advisory Group to the Ministry of Health in New Zealand. The Gap Analysis in New Zealand showed wide national variation in availability of palliative care physicians and highlighted their recruitment and retention as the biggest issue for the future.[38] Haematology services are variably integrated within cancer services, while there is a national or state-wide approach to paediatric and adolescent/young adult services. Both countries have government-controlled pharmaceutical budgets, but differ in medications funded in public hospitals, e.g. cetuximab and bevacizumab are approved for colorectal cancer in Australia but not New Zealand. Although all the cancer plans support research, funding for academic trials is declining.

Acute oncology services in Australasia have been transformed over the last decade, with an increased focus on the patient and greater equality of access. The details of services still vary between states and networks, although the aims are similar. However, significant challenges remain in serving remote populations, and in meeting the needs of the growing and increasingly aging population with greater comorbidity. New models of care with creative use of the workforce and new technologies are being evolved in both countries.

Further reading

1   *Australian Bureau of Statistics [Internet]. Population by Age and Sex, Regions of Australia, 2011*, cat. no. 3235.0. Main Features. [updated 12 Sep 2012, cited 26 Sep 2012]. Canberra: Australian Bureau of Statistics; c.2012. Available from: www.abs.gov.au/Ausstats/abs@.nsf/mf/3235.0

2   Australian Bureau of Statistics [Internet]. *Population Distribution, Aboriginal and Torres Strait Islander Australians, 2006*, cat. no. 4705.0. [updated 18 Jun 2012, cited 26 Sep 2012]. Canberra: Australian Bureau of Statistics; c.2007. Available from: www.abs.gov.au/Ausstats/abs@.nsf/mf/4705.0

3   Geoscience Australia [Internet]. *Area of Australia – States and Territories.* [updated 18 Nov 2010, cited 26 Sep 2012]. Canberra: Geoscience Australia; c.2010. Available from: www.ga.gov.au/education/geoscience-basics/dimensions/area-of-australia-states-and-territories.html

4   Macdonald, T, Worsfold, C, Weir, R. *Cancer in the South Island of New Zealand: Health Needs Assessment – 2010.* Christchurch: Southern Cancer Network; July 2010. 94pp.

5   Northern Cancer Network [Internet]. Auckland: Northern Cancer Network; c.2008–13. Available from: www.northerncancernetwork.org.nz

6   Midland Cancer Network [Internet]. Hamilton: Midland Cancer Network; c.2013. Available from: www.midlandcancernetwork.org.nz

7   Central Cancer Network [Internet]. Palmerston North: Central Cancer Network; c.2013.
    Available from: www.centralcancernetwork.org.nz

8   Southern Cancer Network [Internet]. Christchurch: Southern Cancer Network; 2013.
    www.southerncancernetwork.org.nz

9   Australian Institute of Health and Welfare [Internet]. *Australian Cancer Incidence and
    Mortality (ACIM) Books.* [updated 11 Dec 2012], Canberra: Australian Institute of Health and
    Welfare; c.2013. Available from: www.aihw.gov.au/acim-books

10 Ministry of Health. *Cancer: New Registrations and Deaths 2009.* Wellington: Ministry of
    Health; July 2012.

11 Royal Australian and New Zealand College of Radiologists. Linear Accelerator Fleet in 2012.
    In: *Planning for the Best: Tripartite National Strategic Plan for Radiation Oncology 2012-2022,
    version 1.* Sydney; Wellington: Royal Australian and New Zealand College of Radiologists; 20
    Jun 2012. 136pp.

12 Iain Ward, personal communication, 10 August 2012.

13 Blinman PL, Grimison P, Barton MB *et al.* The shortage of medical oncologists: the
    Australian Medical Oncologist Workforce Study. *Med J Aust* 2012; **196**: 58–61.

14 Australian Institute of Health and Welfare. *Medical labour force 2007. National health labour
    force series no. 44.* Cat. no. HWL 45. Canberra: Australian Institute of Health and Welfare; Oct
    2009. 72pp.

15 Cranleigh Health. *Report to the Ministry of Health: New models of care for medical oncology.*
    Auckland: Cranleigh Health; 5 Oct 2011. 120pp. Available from:
    www.midlandcancernetwork.org.nz/file/fileid/41071

16 Leung, J, Vukolova, N; Faculty of Radiation Oncology, RANZCR. Faculty of Radiation
    Oncology 2010 workforce survey. *J Med Imaging Radiat Oncol* 2011; **55**: 622–32.

17 Underhill CR, Goldstein D, Grogan PB. Inequity in rural cancer survival in Australia is not an
    insurmountable problem. *Med J Australia* 2006; **185**: 479–80.

18 Anderiesz, C, Elwood, M, Hill, D. Commentary: Cancer control policy in Australia. *Aust New
    Zealand Health Policy* 2006; **3**: 12.

19 Adams, P, Hardwick, J, Embree, V, Sinclair, S, Conn, B, Bishop, J. *Literature review: Models of
    cancer services for rural and remote communities.* Sydney: Cancer Institute NSW; March 2009.

20 Hill, S, Sarfati, D, Blakely, T, *et al.* Ethnicity and management of colon cancer in New
    Zealand: do indigenous patients get a worse deal? *Cancer* 2010; **116**: 3205–14.

21 Underhill, C, Bartel, R, Goldstein, D, i Mapping oncology services in regional and rural
    Australia. *Aust J Rural Health* 2009; **17**: 321–9.

22 Clinical Oncological Society of Australia, The Cancer Council Australia and the National
    Cancer Control Initiative. *Optimising Cancer Care in Australia.* Melbourne: National Cancer
    Control Initiative; Feb 2003. 122pp.

23 Cancer Australia [Internet]. Surry Hills, NSW: Cancer Australia; c.2013. Available from:
    www.canceraustralia.gov.au

24 Cancer Control New Zealand [Internet]. Wellington: Cancer Control New Zealand; 2013.
    Available from: www.cancercontrolnz.govt.nz

25 Barton, M, Frommer, M, Olver, I, *et al.* A Cancer Services Framework for Victoria and future
    directions for the Peter MacCallum Cancer Institute. Final Report. Melbourne: Department of
    Health; Jul 2003. 135pp.

26 Cancer Institute NSW. *NSW Cancer plan 2004–06.* Sydney: The Cancer Institute; Jul 2004. 116pp. Available from: www.cancerinstitute.org.au/publications/i/nsw-cancer-plan-2004-06

27 Dalton, L, Luxford, K, Boyle, F, Goldstein, D, Underhill, C, Yates, P. An educational workshop program for rural practitioners to encourage best practice for delivery of systemic adjuvant therapy. *J Cancer Educ* 2006; **21**: 35–9.

28 Koczwara, B, Francis, K, Marine, F, Goldstein, D, Underhill, C, Olver, I. Reaching further with Online education? The development of an effective Online programme in palliative oncology. *J Cancer Educ* 2010; **25**: 317–23.

29 Cancer Institute NSW [Internet]. *EviQ: Cancer Treatments Online.* Sydney: Cancer Institute NSW; c.2012. Available from: www.eviq.org.au

30 Olver, I, Shepherd, L, Selva-Nayagam, S. Beyond the bush telegraph: telehealth for remote cancer control and support. *Cancer Forum* 2007; **31**: 77–80.

31 Grimison, P, Phillips, P, Butow, P, *et al.* Are visiting oncologists enough? A qualitative study of the needs of Australian rural and regional cancer patients, carers and health professionals. *Asia Pac J Clin Oncol* 2012. [Epub ahead of print] doi:10.1111/ajco.12014

32 Australian Institute of Health and Welfare 2012. Cancer survival and prevalence in Australia: period estimates from 1982 to 2010. Cancer series no. 69. Cat no. CAN65. Canberra: AIHW.

33 Australian Institute of Health and Welfare. *Cancer incidence projections: Australia, 2011 to 2020. Cancer series no. 66.* Cat no. CAN 62. Canberra: Australian Institute of Health and Welfare; 9 Mar 2012.

34 Ministry of Health. *Medical Oncology National Implementation Plan 2012/13.* Wellington: Ministry of Health; 2012.

35 Southern Cancer Network [Internet]. South Island Clinical Cancer Information System (SICCIS). Christchurch: Southern Cancer Network; 2013. [cited 25 Sep 2012]. Available from: www.southerncancernetwork.org.nz/page/pageid/2145861494

36 Leung, J. The role of the radiation oncologist in systemic therapy – an Australian and New Zealand perspective. *J Nucl Med Radiat Ther* 2012; **S6**: 006.

37 Palliative Care Australia. *Standards for providing quality palliative care for all Australians.* Canberra: Palliative Care Australia; May 2005. 40pp.

38 Ministry of Health. *Gap Analysis of Specialist Palliative Care in New Zealand. Providing a national overview of hospice and hospital-based services.* Wellington: Ministry of Health; Dec 2009.

10 Acute Oncology in a District Hospital – the Airedale Perspective

S Michael Crawford, Patricia Dyminski, Maxine Armitage

Case History

Patient 1.

A 56-year-old man was admitted to the emergency department (ED) with seizures following a fall. At the time he was on chemotherapy for small cell lung cancer with metastases in bone, liver and brain. He was complaining of severe pain in his hip; a subsequent radiograph showed a fractured pelvis. The acute cancer team were paged and asked for advice. A senior nurse and a consultant medical oncologist attended the emergency department.

Patient 2.

A 79-year-old woman was admitted to the emergency department (ED) with abdominal pain. She had cancer of unknown primary and was beyond the active management phase of her cancer journey. The acute cancer team were contacted for advice by pager.

Patient 3.

A 77-year-old man received his third cycle of docetaxel chemotherapy for metastatic carcinoma of the prostate and felt unwell two days later over the weekend. He did not use the 24-hour contact line, but instead telephoned the out-of-hours general practitioner (GP) who gave him oral antibiotics. On Monday morning his family made use of the contact line to telephone the day unit, and were advised by nursing staff to bring him in for urgent assessment. He arrived within 40 minutes of the call.

How were the patients managed?

How has the long-term presence of a resident oncology team promoted acute oncology care?

Background

Cancer care in Airedale Hospital has been provided by resident consultant oncologists and an oncology team for many years. This contrasts with historical arrangements in acute general hospitals (AGHs), where specialist oncology services were largely provided by doctors based in tertiary centres who visited AGHs. It therefore gives us the opportunity to evaluate the impact of this arrangement on acute oncology practice over a lengthy time period.[1,2] The Airedale oncology service came about because in the late 1980s a local cancer research charity, which was seeking to enhance its clinical role, funded a medical oncologist in the hospital. The current oncology team includes two consultants and a trained associate specialist, plus two other specialty doctors employed by Airedale. This team works with four consultants and an associate specialist who are based in the neighbouring Bradford Teaching Hospitals Foundation Trust where the designated inpatient service is located, although most local patients are admitted to Airedale. This arrangement permits a high level of cancer site specialization.

How were the patients managed?

Patient 1 had had a recent CT scan which showed progressive disease, and the patient was due in the outpatient clinic that week for a consultation on the findings, so a decision to discontinue treatment was discussed with the patient in the emergency department. As a surgical approach was not appropriate, this discussion centred on specialist palliative care management. The palliative care team within the hospital was contacted (the community team were already supporting the family at home) and a placement was found for the patient in his chosen hospice. The hospice was out of the local area but appropriate for continued family support. The patient was given adequate analgesia prior to the 30 minute transfer to the hospice direct from the ED.

Patient 2 was assessed in the ED – it was felt acute admission was not appropriate nor in the patient's best interest. The team liaised with the local hospice and the patient was transferred there directly from the ED. She died peacefully there eight days later.

On arrival in the chemotherapy day unit, **patient 3** was lethargic and looked pale and unwell. Within a few minutes of being taken into a room he had collapsed. He was hypotensive, tachycardic and pyrexial. The patient was moved into the dedicated triage room, given intravenous antibiotics (within 1 h of arrival), gelatin infusion, oxygen and all supportive care. The neutrophil count was 0.46×10^9/l. He was kept under special observation in the triage room until a high-dependency bed was made available some six hours later, and he remained there for a week. The patient recovered fully and was discharged 14 days after admission.

The three elements of acute oncology

1) Patients with an established diagnosis of cancer

When such patients develop symptoms which are due to their cancer, they may require admission to hospital for immediate relief and planning of further management. This may be pre-empted if the GP is consulted and a referral to the appropriate site specialist oncology clinic is made, but if this is not achieved the acute oncology service should optimize their care.

We have developed a procedure where the electronic patient administration system of the hospital is used to compare the list of inpatients with the list of those patients who have a history of attendances to oncology clinics. When an individual appears on both lists, the doctor responsible for reviewing the acute oncology service each day ascertains the reason for the patient's admission and offers input into the clinical management. This may involve initiating inpatient investigations, arranging them as an outpatient, or, if the patient's condition is such that it is unlikely that active treatment would be of value, advise that investigation is inappropriate and relevant symptomatic care can be established. In this respect, the close association of the hospital's palliative care team with the acute oncology service is paramount, and is illustrated in the case of patient 2.

2) Acute complications of the systemic treatment of cancer

Principal among these are neutropenia and sepsis, although thrombocytopenia and bleeding, intractable nausea and vomiting, and intractable diarrhoea are all common reasons to come into hospital. In the UK, the care of patients on systemic anticancer treatment has received much attention in recent years, with an enquiry into patients dying within 30 days of chemotherapy identifying that such patients may not be well managed.[3] This enquiry highlighted the fact that management must not rely on patients' strict observance of advice they may receive about who to contact and when. This is illustrated in the case of patient 3.

An active approach to the identification and management of such patients has always been a part of the Airedale Hospital service. The electronic system which identifies patients with an oncological history that are admitted to hospital, and the policy that the Medical Assessment Unit (MAU) is visited each day by a member of the oncology team, ensures that such patients are seen promptly and that there are discussions between the oncology team and the acute medical staff responsible for their care. Haematological patients are admitted directly under the care of a specialist haematologist.

The development of oral chemotherapeutic agents has thrown up an important issue. On a busy acute medical unit, cancer patients very often have their long-term medication continued while their reason for admission is being evaluated and treated. This creates the danger of continuing an oral chemotherapeutic agent in a patient suffering adverse effects from that treatment.[4] Input from the acute oncology team into such patients' management ensures that this treatment is stopped when it is appropriate to do so.

3) New diagnosis of cancer

At Airedale, a medical oncology opinion could always be sought early in the diagnostic process; the advent of the formal acute oncology service has led to this being refined.

The first area of refinement is to avoid patients with early or newly diagnosed cancer being admitted to the ED. The ambiguous symptoms with which patients with early cancers may present mean that a GP may find it difficult to identify the right specialty when directing a referral. The acute oncology service now provides a clinic where a GP can use a specific fast-track form to make a referral without having to identify a primary site; such patients usually have their initial contact as either a clinic appointment or a CT scan within a week of the referral. This enables the requirements of the National Institute for Health and Care Excellence (NICE) guidance on malignancy of unknown origin to be met in a timely manner.[5] It marks a necessary departure from medical oncologists' traditional perspective that, as a tertiary specialty, they should only see patients with a confirmed diagnosis. There is a need to exercise discretion in accepting patients to this service in order to avoid running an old-fashioned general medical clinic, but a conversation with the referring GP is helpful in ensuring appropriateness.

Referral to this clinic also facilitates the early discharge of patient whose cancer is diagnosed after an acute admission.

The role of nurses in acute oncology

The doctor's role in the acute oncology service is shared among six individuals. This carries the risk of discontinuity of care, but this is bridged by the fact that a senior oncology nurse, one of two, accompanies the medical oncologist during the initial visit.

In fact, the nurse may already have undertaken a preliminary assessment. The oncology nurses also ensure that a patient's needs are followed up appropriately throughout their stay, with the doctors' involvement not always necessary. This team ensures that the specialty view is communicated to the ward medical and nursing teams, with specific nursing issues discussed within that profession.

This role extends beyond the wards. The proactive approach of nurses has, in the words of an ED consultant, 'driven the awareness' of staff who discuss cancer patients with the appropriate clinical colleagues. This may result in the appropriate arrangements being made for an admission or, preferably, appropriate outpatient attendances may be arranged with the oncology team. Follow-up telephone calls are made by nurses to patients who are sent home from the ED. As a consequence, the nurses are the first persons the ward staff think of to seek advice. The ED is often the place where the decision not to admit a patient to hospital can be made if the cancer does not warrant active management and where an appropriate alternative is available. The three case histories above show how interaction with the hospice sector can achieve this.

The, oncology nurses, with advanced training and extensive experience, also have a special role in providing education – including mandatory training – to junior doctors, ED and MAU personnel.

Conclusion

The place of oncology in the body politic

Integration of medical oncology into the services of Airedale Hospital has meant that the oncological perspective can be represented at the in-house educational meetings. The collaboration of oncology with other disciplines is recognized as being invaluable to the ethos of the modern AGH and involves participation in the administrative structure of the hospital, including representation on relevant committees. The value of this was recognized in the National Cancer Action Group report, but is clearly absent when the oncology service is only provided by a series of transient visiting doctors. This applies to all aspects of oncology, but it is especially important in the acute area, where issues cannot be covered by site-specific specialty meetings. These relationships can be cemented by involvement in the social aspects of the hospital's wider team; this is harder if the doctor's presence is transient. The importance from the patient's point of view of the service being within the local hospital must be recognized.

Acute oncology is developing in the UK as a recommended remedy for some of the deficiencies of the nation's cancer services that have recently been recognized. Very few institutions have developed such services over time as in Airedale Hospital. Trainee oncologists have little exposure to daily life in an AGH, since most of the training occurs either in specialized hospitals or in specialized departments within institutions, which are extremely large by international standards. It will be important in the coming years to inculcate an understanding and enthusiasm for all aspects of oncology in the acute general hospital.

Further reading

1   National Chemotherapy Advisory Group. *Chemotherapy Services in England: Ensuring quality and safety.* London: Department of Health; 21 Aug 2009. 70pp.

2   King J, Ingham-Clark C, Parker C, Jennings R, Leonard P. Towards saving a million bed days: reducing length of stay through an acute oncology model of care for inpatients diagnosed as having cancer. *BMJ Qual Saf* 2011; **20**: 718–24.

3   Mort D, Lansdown M, Smith N, Protopapa K, Mason M. *For better, for worse? A review of the care of patients who died within 30 days of receiving systemic anti-cancer therapy.* London: National Confidential Enquiry into Patient Outcome and Death (NCEPOD); Nov 2008. 150pp.

4   Booth JA, Booth C, Crawford SM. Inappropriate continuation of medication when patients are admitted acutely: the example of capecitabine. *Clin Med* 2011; **11**: 511.

5   National Institute for Health and Clinical Excellence [Internet]. *Metastatic malignant disease of unknown primary origin (CG104).* London: National Institute for Health and Care Excellence. c.2010. Available from: www.nice.org.uk/CG104

11 The Future of Acute Oncology

Alison Young, Ernie Marshall

The National Chemotherapy Advisory Group (NCAG) report in 2009 outlined a number of recommendations aimed at improving the safety and quality of chemotherapy services in England and Wales. Among these was a statement that all acute trusts with an emergency department should develop an acute oncology service (AOS). A potential model of care was described that included five sessions of consultant oncology time and one full-time equivalent nurse specialist. Thus, the concept of 'acute oncology' was born. From the outset, the emphasis of acute oncology was driven by safety and quality of care for inpatients, although complex service configurations and commissioning have proved to be major challenges. Preliminary surveys in 2011/12 have demonstrated widespread implementation of AOS, with many new initiatives that go beyond the original NCAG model and which illustrate an ever greater potential for service improvement and redesign.[1]

Acute oncology represents a major shift in the direction of oncology from an ever greater need for subspecialties and personalized medicine back towards a need to deliver unplanned oncology care using basic cross-cutting principles that are relevant to all cancer patients. Evidence, albeit largely anecdotal, suggests that acute oncology has been warmly welcomed by NHS trusts and general medical colleagues, and is leading not only to improved care and coordination, but also to a reduction in length of hospital stay and efficiency savings. It is also important to recognise that acute oncology will affect the way cancer medicine is delivered throughout the world, not just in the UK.

The future challenge of acute oncology remains significant. However, there are also huge opportunities for acute oncology teams (AOTs) to engage with and influence therapeutic strategies that allow the integration of highly specialized cancer treatment alongside local delivery and admission avoidance. In this vision, AOTs will have a leading role to play in service development alongside partner organizations in both secondary and primary care.

Admission avoidance

Inpatient care has been a major focus for AOTs, but it is clear that future healthcare strategy is towards self-care, early intervention and community-based services. In England and Wales, the NHS Confederation believes that at least 25% of patients in hospital beds could be looked after by NHS staff at home. In this respect, future AOS will need to embrace a wide range of admission avoidance strategies, as illustrated in Figure 11.1

Decision making and patient and professional information

Future care will require greater contingency emergency planning, and greater access to information and advice to support patients and professionals; this will enable early detection and management of cancer complications. Developments of existing triage, patient-held records, timely access to summary oncology dashboards and innovation in information technology (e.g. smart-phone applications, or 'apps') will all improve

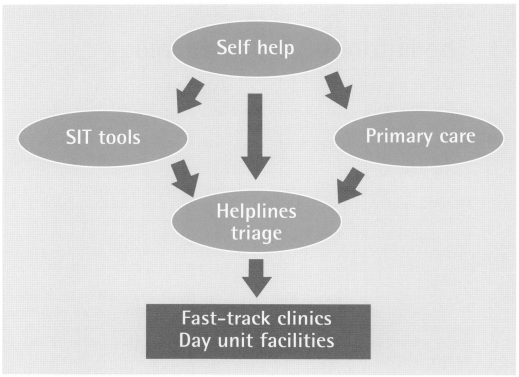

Figure 11.1 **Strategies to avoid admission**

opportunities to reduce the need for hospital attendance.[2] For example, future management of suspected febrile neutropenia might incorporate community-based services that allow rapid assessment of neutrophil count, risk stratification and early antibiotic, all coordinated through acute oncology triage. In this scenario, only the most serious cases may require hospital intervention.

The ageing population

As the population in the developed world ags, larger amounts of healthcare expenditure will need to be focused on elderly people. Growing numbers of elderly people will naturally have an impact on the number of inpatient care episodes and hence the investigation of patients with suspected cancer. Acute oncology services will need to be able to handle the likely increase in diagnostic and clinical events in this expanding elderly population, both in hospital and in the community.

Improving access to acute oncology services

It is vital that AOS in the future are developed to improve access to cancer services, facilitating timely diagnosis and management of suspected cancers. Inevitably, this is likely to generate pressure on healthcare providers, as patients who are in the early access models (being encouraged by the awareness campaigns to go and see their GP) will also have some impact on immediate early diagnostic services. As we move towards strategies in healthcare that will diagnose cancer patients earlier, we are likely to generate a population of patients with increasing uncertainty who will require prompt access to the appropriate diagnostic support services and specialists. This is an area upon which acute oncology is likely to need to focus. Although some of these patients will enter surgical diagnostic pathways, others will almost certainly require oncological input early on in their diagnostic pathway.

Access to outpatient fast-track clinics

Many patients will continue to require assessment by oncology teams despite enhanced information and community support. Consequently, access to fast-track clinics and day unit review will become ever more relevant. Increasingly, these outpatient services will need to incorporate extended hours of work, and provide facilities to support ambulatory care and day procedures that have historically required inpatient stay. These services will need to integrate with and work alongside existing acute medical and palliative care services as a means of maximising opportunities for efficiency and team working, thus avoiding acute cancer services working in isolation. Capacity will continue to be a significant challenge that will only be met by developing allied work streams in community chemotherapy and devolved follow-up for low-risk patients.

Community-based oncology

Non-surgical oncology has been viewed as a specialist tertiary service for many years and will continue to require subspecialist expertise in the context of multidisciplinary team working and personalized medicine. Despite this, there are many opportunities to develop community work streams that allow oncology to engage with primary care services in the local cancer network, with the aim of promoting self-help, holistic care and an element of follow-up, in a manner analogous to other chronic disease states. Acute oncology teams are uniquely placed to lead on this important area of service development and to influence primary care cancer strategy. Indeed, in the future, AOTs may be best placed working across the hospital and community interface in close collaboration with palliative care and community key workers.

Training and research

Acute oncology teams have a critical role to play in delivering training and education to all professionals who respond to patients with cancer and acute cancer needs. Solutions will include generic training at all levels of education, but also the development of innovative e-learning modules and the evolution of acute oncology link-staff with the responsibility of disseminating acute oncology information and principles of care to the wider NHS community. In the hospital setting, the care of critically ill cancer patients may evolve a degree of acute oncology subspecialization and the emergence of a much-needed research and evidence base in this orphan area. High-quality research in the field of acute oncology is severely lacking and will pose a significant challenge in protocol development and delivery, but it remains an important future direction for AOTs in the developed world.

Service configuration

The National Confidential Enquiry into Patient Outcome and Death (NCEPOD) and NCAG reports highlight the fragmentation of care that has emerged, in part due to the greater subspecialization within oncology and the lack of focus on emergency cancer patient pathways in England and Wales. Not infrequently, the delivery of specialist care is dislocated from the patient pathway that is required to manage acute complications, and is often characterized by poor communication. Developments within acute oncology have often illustrated the benefit of teamwork across general medical disciplines and the importance of expert oncology provision beyond the cancer centre. Acute oncology nurses often represent the first point of contact and offer a potential model to develop acute oncology nurse-led services. The NCAG recommended five sessions of consultant medical time to serve as a potential model, but this remains fluid and dependent upon local service configuration. Irrespective of the model, and accepting that models will be different throughout the developed world, it remains essential that strong clinical leadership supports the acute oncology concept if the full potential of AOS is to be realized.

Within the NHS specifically, the model of future cancer service provision must respond to the challenge of personalized medicine, subspecialization and acute oncology. This may signal a movement towards a more devolved acute general oncology provision supporting common cancer care, and a second tier of centralized subspecialist services. Oncologists may continue to work across these interfaces, or increasingly work within a specific area of expertise.

Should AOS develop a defined inpatient bed base? The NCAG report envisaged that acute oncology would be a consultation service that would not require inpatient beds. This vision supports the concept of admission avoidance and the aim of reducing the total hospital bed stock, but there remains a case for a more centralized approach to inpatient care for cancer patients that could result in improved coordination of care and improved clinical leadership.

Funding acute oncology services

Acute oncology services aim to improve patient safety, quality and coordination of care; thus, funding was anticipated to arise from efficiency savings. Although this approach has enabled many NHS trusts to develop acute oncology provision, it is clear that efficiency savings alone will not support the natural evolution and growth of future AOS. Commissioners need to recognize that future developments will require funding to cover the activities of the AOS, ensuring that they are high quality. There may well be a shift from traditional funding streams towards the support for innovative outpatient therapies and diagnostic and management procedures

Conclusion

The increasing incidence of cancer, the explosion of new therapies, and the apparent tension between greater site specialization and devolved care will continue to challenge healthcare service configuration. Against this backdrop, acute oncology represents a key service development that will remain at the forefront of cancer strategy. The future challenge for acute oncology rests with its ability to develop responsive pathways that increasingly inform patients and professionals alike, enhance opportunities for community care, and provide speedy access to advice and clinical review '24 hours a day, 7 days per week'.[1]

Further reading

1 National Chemotherapy Advisory Group. *Developing an Acute Oncology service: concepts and case studies.* London: National Cancer Action Team; 29 Mar 2012. 32pp. Available from: http://ncat.nhs.uk/news-and-events/developing-acute-oncology-service

2 Royal College of Physicians and Royal College of Radiologists. *Cancer patients in crisis: responding to urgent needs.* Report of a working party. London: Royal College of Physicians; Nov 2012. 114pp.

Complications of Systemic Therapy

12 Febrile Neutropenia

Amy Ford, Ernie Marshall

Case Histories

Two patients present directly to the oncology centre with fever. The salient features are as follows:

Patient 1: A 22-year-old man with no comorbidities has recorded a temperature of 38.0°C at home 12 days after his first cycle of adjuvant chemotherapy for testicular cancer. He feels well and has no localizing symptoms.

Vital signs for **patient 1** read: temperature 38.0°C, pulse 80 bpm, blood pressure 125/80 mmHg. A full blood count reveals: Hb 10.1 g/dl; WBC 1 ×10⁹/l; neutrophils 0.4 × 10⁹/l; platelets 200 × 10⁹/l.

Patient 2: A 63-year-old man is known to have chronic obstructive pulmonary disease (COPD). He is unwell and dehydrated seven days after his third cycle of palliative chemotherapy for bowel cancer. Vital signs: temperature 38.8°C, pulse 124 bpm, blood pressure 110/70 mmHg. Full blood count reveals: Hb 9.2 g/dl; WBC 0.5 × 10⁹/l; neutrophils 0.08×10⁹/l; platelets 100×10⁹/l.

Subsequently, you receive a call from the local district general hospital (DGH) regarding an oncology patient who has presented with fever to the emergency department (ED), and you are asked to advise. A summary of the verbal report is as follows:

Patient 3: A 52-year-old woman, with a peripherally inserted central catheter (PICC) line *in situ* has presented with a history of rigors nine days after her fourth cycle of adjuvant chemotherapy for breast cancer. She has been receiving primary prophylaxis with pegfilgrastim after each cycle, to reduce the risk of neutropenia. Vital signs: temperature 36.8°C, pulse 112 bpm, blood pressure 90/unrecordable mmHg. A full blood count reveals: Hb 8.9 g/dl; WBC 0.7×10⁹/l; neutrophils 0.1 × 10⁹; platelets 120 × 10⁹/l.

What is febrile neutropenia?

How do you evaluate febrile neutropenia?

How would you assess and manage each of these patients?

Background

What is febrile neutropenia?

Febrile neutropenia is defined as a temperature of greater than 38°C, with a neutrophil count <0.5 × 10⁹/l in a patient undergoing anticancer treatment, most commonly cytotoxic chemotherapy.[1] Newer, biological systemic anticancer treatments and radiotherapy have a much lower propensity to cause neutropenia. Haematological malignancies have a relatively high rate of febrile neutropenia. Febrile neutropenia is a significant cause of cancer-related mortality, with the number of attributable deaths doubling between 2001 and 2010, even after adjusting for the increasing number of cancers diagnosed during this time period.[1] The majority of febrile neutropenic deaths are in those aged 65–79 years. The explanation for the rising mortality is unclear, but may be related to the increasing use of chemotherapy, greater dose intensity, the treatment of patients who would previously have been considered too high risk for chemotherapy, and the increase in antibiotic resistance. The National Confidential Enquiry into Patient Outcome and Death (NCEPOD) report into patient deaths within 30 days of receiving systemic anti cancer therapy also found evidence of increasing dislocation of care, and deemed the management of febrile neutropenia unsatisfactory.[2]

The pattern of causative organisms in febrile neutropenia has changed from being largely gram-negative pathogens during the early years of chemotherapy use, to predominantly gram-positive organisms since the introduction of indwelling plastic catheters in the 1980s, which promote the colonization and entry of gram-positive skin flora into the bloodstream.[3] Gram-positive cocci causing febrile neutropenia include *Staphylococcus epidermidis*, *Staph. aureus* and streptococci.[4] Drug-resistant gram-positive organisms, such as methicillin-resistant *Staph. aureus* (MRSA) and vancomycin-resistant *Enterococcus* (VRE) are increasingly prevalent. Gram-negative organisms are also implicated in febrile neutropenia, in particular *Klebsiella* species and *Escherichia coli* strains, among which antibiotic resistance due to extended-spectrum β-lactamase (ESBL) production is increasing.[3]

There is evidence that primary antibiotic prophylaxis, most commonly with a quinolone or cotrimoxazole, reduces the incidence of febrile neutropenia and short-term mortality.[5] However, this needs to be balanced against the risks of increasing antibiotic resistance and the adverse effects of antibiotic use. The National Institute for Health and Care Excellence (NICE) guidelines recommend the use of prophylactic quinolones for the predicted duration of neutropenia only in patients being treated for acute leukaemias, stem cell transplants, or solid tumours where significant neutropenia (neutrophil count $< 0.5 \times 10^9$/l) is anticipated.[1]

The severity and duration of neutropenia can be moderated with primary prophylaxis using granulocyte colony-stimulating factor (G-CSF). Although there is no convincing evidence that prophylaxis with G-CSF reduces short-term mortality, it has been shown to reduce the rate of febrile neutropenia and shorten the length of hospital stay, which may help maintain the dose intensity of chemotherapy used with curative intent.[6] The efficacy of G-CSF may vary according to the type of cancer therapy (leukaemia, lymphoma/solid tumour, stem cell transplant), and must be weighed against the side effects of its use, such as bone pain, headache and nausea. There is some evidence that pegylated G-CSF (pegfilgrastim), which requires less frequent administration, is more effective in preventing febrile neutropenia than the unpegylated form (filgrastim).[6] NICE guidelines advocate against the routine use of G-CSF, unless it is an integral part of a specific chemotherapy regimen. International guidelines recommend the use of G-CSF in selected patients with a risk of febrile neutropenia exceeding 20%.[7,8]

How do you evaluate febrile neutropenia?

Patients who present with a fever following anticancer treatment should be promptly assessed with a thorough history and examination, having particular regard to any potential focus of infection. The possibility of cellulitis, abscesses and infections of the oral cavity should not be overlooked. Investigations should include full blood count (FBC), renal function, liver function, C-reactive protein, lactate and blood cultures. Where a central venous catheter is in use, peripheral blood cultures should be obtained in addition. Urinalysis, chest X-ray, stool, sputum and cerebrospinal fluid culture should only be undertaken when clinically indicated. The differential diagnoses to be considered include malignancy-related fever, pulmonary embolism, and chemotherapy-induced fever (most commonly seen with bleomycin). Because of the potential risks of missing the diagnosis of febrile neutropenia, any fever in a patient undergoing chemotherapy should be treated as septic in origin until proved otherwise. All hospitals with an emergency department (ED) should ensure that links are established with local acute oncology services (AOS) to facilitate the development of a febrile neutropenia management pathway, which should incorporate early review by a member of the oncology team.[9]

Only a minority of patients will develop life-threatening infections or suffer other serious complications, and there is increasingly a shift towards the stratification of patients with febrile neutropenia between those at high and low risk of septic complications. Risk stratification reduces the length of hospitalization and prevents overtreating those at low risk. Stratification is based on presenting signs and symptoms, the nature of the underlying malignancy, and existing comorbidities, and should be undertaken using a validated risk scoring tool, such as the Multinational Association of Supportive Care in Cancer (MASCC) risk index.[10,11]

Table 12.1 Multinational Association of Supportive Care in Cancer (MASCC) Index	
Characteristic burden of illness:	Score
Either no or mild symptoms*	5
Or moderate symptoms*	3
No hypotension	5
No chronic obstructive pulmonary disease	4
Solid tumour/lymphoma or no previous fungal infection	4
No dehydration	3
Outpatient status at onset of fever	3
Age <60 years	2

* Points attributable to burden of illness are not cumulative. The maximal theoretical score is therefore 26. A threshold ≥21 points defines 'low risk'.

The burden of illness (the first characteristic in the risk index) represents a measure of how unwell the patient is at presentation, but lacks objective definition. Clinical experience is needed to inform this judgement and it is recommended that risk stratification be undertaken by a healthcare professional with experience in managing the complications of anticancer treatment.[1]

Low-risk patients should be considered for treatment with oral antibiotics, followed by early discharge after taking into account their social circumstances. The minimum safe period of observation prior to discharge has yet to be determined, but most studies to date have observed patients for at least 24 hours prior to discharge.[3] Intravenous antibiotics are warranted if coexisting complications of chemotherapy, such as vomiting or severe mucositis, prevent the administration of oral medication. High-risk patients should receive empirical intravenous antibiotics as soon as possible. A national target time of one hour has been set from the point at which a likely diagnosis of febrile neutropenia is made (based on clinical assessment rather than laboratory results) to administration of antibiotic therapy.[12]

When choosing empirical antibiotics, the epidemiological spectrum of bloodstream isolates and regional patterns of antibiotic resistance should be considered. Treatment should follow local guidelines. In the absence of patient-specific or local microbiological contraindications, NICE guidance recommends β-lactam monotherapy using piperacillin/tazobactam combination antibiotic as initial empirical treatment, and advises against the use of aminoglycosides in this context, as there is no evidence that combined therapy reduces mortality. Monotherapy is also associated with fewer adverse effects, e.g. nephrotoxicity, and avoids the need to monitor aminoglycoside levels.[1] Antibiotics should be discontinued in patients whose febrile neutropenia has responded to treatment, as evidenced by lysis of fever and subjective and objective improvement, irrespective of neutrophil count.[1] Where an organism has been isolated, treatment should be continued for a minimum of five days.

Persistent fever, in the absence of clinical deterioration or new focal signs, is not an indication for switching antibiotic therapy unless guided by culture results.[1,3] In the absence of a source of bacterial infection, patients with a persistent fever after 4–7 days who are expected to be neutropenic for longer than seven days should be considered for empirical antifungal therapy and investigated for invasive fungal infections.[3] Choice of empirical antifungal agent, if indicated, will depend on whether or not the patient has already received prophylactic antifungal treatment.[3]

How would you assess and manage each of these patients?

Patient 1:

This man is febrile on day 13 following chemotherapy. Assessment using the MASCC index (Table 12.1) stratifies him as being at low risk of septic complications, with a score of 26 (mild symptoms = 5; no hypotension = 5; no COPD = 4; solid tumour = 4; no dehydration = 3; outpatient = 3; age <60 years = 2). Peripheral blood cultures should be taken. Urinalysis, stool and sputum cultures, and chest X-ray are only necessary if clinically indicated by the history or physical examination. It would be appropriate to treat this patient with empirical oral antibiotics, as per local guidelines, but would not be unreasonable to wait for the results of initial investigations rather than initiating treatment immediately. In units lacking familiarity with risk stratification, commencing intravenous antibiotics – with subsequent stepdown to oral antibiotics after review by the acute oncology team – would also be an option. If this patient has a good understanding of the risks of febrile neutropenia, is compliant with treatment, lives with a responsible adult and can easily return to hospital in the event of complications, he could be considered for early discharge after 24 hours of clinical observation. It should be emphasized that this patient should have a low threshold for contacting the unit if he has further symptoms.

Patient 2:

This patient is at high risk of septic complications, with a MASCC index score of 10 (moderate symptoms = 3; hypotensive = 0; COPD = 0; solid tumour = 4; dehydrated = 0; outpatient = 3; age >60 years = 0). He should be treated with empirical intravenous antibiotics, as per local guidelines, without delay. Peripheral blood cultures, chest X-ray and other investigations indicated clinically should be undertaken, but these should not delay the first dose of antibiotics. In addition, he requires intravenous fluids and optimization of his COPD. Any other side effects of chemotherapy or the underlying cancer should also be addressed.

The patient should be reviewed daily. Empirical antibiotic treatment should be altered in light of any positive culture results. Persistent fever alone, in the absence of clinical deterioration, is not an indication for changing antibiotics. Intravenous antibiotics may be switched to oral after 48 hours if the risk of developing septic complications is re-assessed, using the MASCC score, as low.[1] Antibiotic treatment can be stopped once the neutropenic sepsis has responded to treatment, irrespective of neutrophil count.[1] It is not uncommon for cultures to yield negative results, and in 70%–80% of cases the infective organism is never confirmed.[3]

Following recovery, the risks and benefits of continuing palliative chemotherapy should be reviewed by the patient's oncologist and discussed with the patient. If chemotherapy is continued, a dose reduction may be considered to reduce the risk of further episodes of febrile neutropenia. In the palliative context, chemotherapy dose reduction would be more appropriate than secondary prophylaxis with G-CSF, because the latter is unlikely to effect clinically important outcomes in this setting.

Patient 3:

This woman is not pyrexial at the time of presentation, but is severely shocked. Classic signs of infection can be diminished in immunosuppressed patients. With the history of recent chemotherapy and rigors she should be assumed to be suffering with neutropenic sepsis until proved otherwise. Rigors may be associated with flushing of the PICC line and enquiry into this should form part of the history taking. In addition, the PICC line should be examined for any signs of inflammation. This patient's MASCC index score is 16 (moderate symptoms = 3; hypotensive = 0; no COPD = 4; solid tumour = 4; dehydrated = 0; outpatient = 3; age <60 years = 2), putting her at high risk of septic complications. Blood cultures should be obtained from the indwelling venous catheter, and also peripherally if possible, but should not delay treatment.

The patient's clinical condition and history warrant fluid resuscitation and treatment with empirical intravenous antibiotics, as per local guidelines, without waiting for confirmation of the neutrophil count. In the absence of obvious infection associated with the indwelling venous catheter, or specific local microbiological indications, empirical glycopeptide antibiotics should not be included in this patient's initial treatment. There is little evidence of increased effectiveness of treatment or any reduction in short-term mortality with the addition of empirical glycopeptide antibiotics in this context, but greater hepatic and nephrotoxicity are recognized consequences.[1] If there is no strong clinical suspicion of central line infection there is no need for its removal in the initial phase of management, but this should be reviewed if there is no resolution of fever or there is evidence of post-flushing fever.[1] Early review by a member of the acute oncology team (AOT) at the DGH should be arranged. This can be facilitated by the development of an electronic system that automatically alerts the AOT of the admission of any patient who has recently received chemotherapy, and by the joint development of integrated care pathways by oncology, haematology and emergency medicine teams. There should be a low threshold for assessment by the intensive care team if there is no response to treatment.

For this patient, who is receiving adjuvant treatment, the balance of risks and benefits of continuing treatment are different than for 'Patient 2' (see above). As she has suffered febrile neutropenia despite the use of primary prophylaxis with G-CSF as an integral part of her chemotherapy regimen, additional secondary prophylaxis with a quinolone may be considered to maintain dose intensity, especially if she has suffered more than one episode of febrile neutropenia.

Recent developments

The NCEPOD report revealed that the management of febrile neutropenia did not meet a consistently high standard across the UK.[2] In addition, it highlighted that a proportion of patients delayed seeking medical advice for at least 24 hours. This has resulted in the evolution of acute oncology services nationally, and the development of a clinical guideline for the prevention and management of neutropenic sepsis by NICE (see Figures 12.1 and 12.2).[1] It has been recommended that all NHS Trusts have policies on the management of febrile neutropenia,[12] and that patients are provided with written information about febrile neutropenia, with advice on when and how to contact 24-hour specialist oncology services.[1] The 'bundle' framework established by the Surviving Sepsis Campaign should be incorporated into care pathways for febrile neutropenia.[13]

Although developed outside of the UK context, the Infectious Diseases Society of America (IDSA) has produced a clinical guideline for the use of antimicrobial agents in neutropenic patients with cancer.[3] Although local patterns of antibiotic resistance and microbiological epidemiology should always be considered in the treatment of febrile neutropenia, much of the evidence and guidance contained within the IDSA guideline is relevant to international practice.

Conclusion

Febrile neutropenia requires prompt diagnosis and treatment with empirical antibiotic treatment, irrespective of where patients present. All hospitals need policies in place for the management of febrile neutropenia to ensure every patient receives the highest standard of care. Risk stratification tools such as the MASCC index are central to avoid overtreating low-risk patients and for freeing up hospital beds by facilitating the early discharge of carefully selected patients, as well as ensuring the early and appropriate treatment of high-risk patients. Clinical experience in the management of febrile neutropenia and risk stratification is vital in ensuring this is done safely, and AOTs therefore have an important role in optimizing the management of febrile neutropenia outside of specialist oncology centres.

Patients need to be provided with print or multimedia information, to ensure they are aware of the signs, symptoms and risks of febrile neutropenia and the need to seek medical advice early. The importance of having access to a thermometer at home should be stressed.

Figure 12.1 Summary of recommendations for prevention and management of neutropenic sepsis in cancer patients. (Adapted from ref.(1) with permission.)

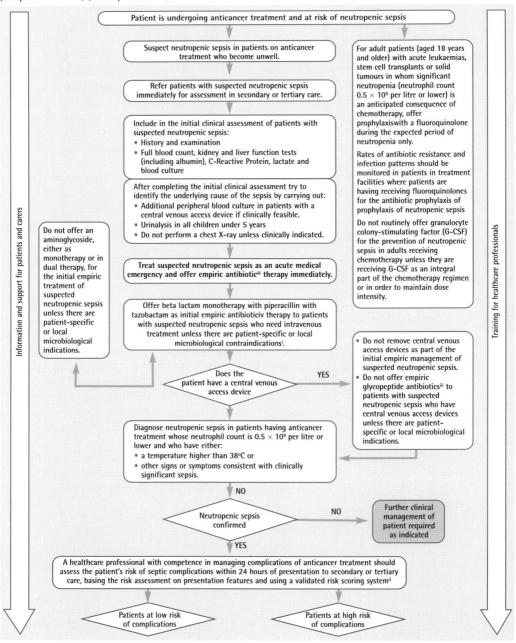

[i] Be sure to note local marketing authorization regarding piperacillin with tazobactam use in children aged under 2 years. The prescriber should follow relevant professional guidance, taking full responsibility for the decision. If required, the child's parent or carer should provide informed consent, which should be documented.

[ii] For example, the Multinational Association of Supportive Care in Cancer (MASCC) risk index. See also Table 12.1.

[iii] An empiric antibiotic is given to a person before a specific microorganism or source of the potential infection is known. It is usually a broad-spectrum antibiotic and the treatment may change if the microorganism or source is confirmed.

Figure 12.2 Overview of low- and high-risk management for cancer patients with confirmed neutropenic sepsis following risk stratification. Adapted from ref.(1) with permission.

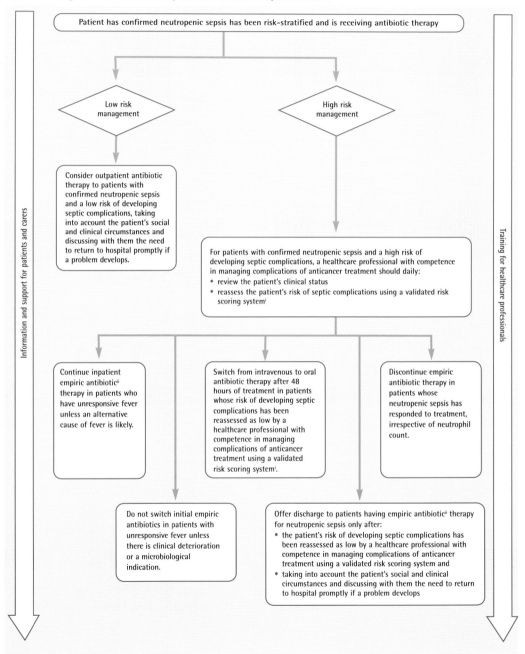

i For example, the Multinational Association of Supportive Care in Cancer (MASCC) risk index. See also Table 12.1.

ii An empiric antibiotic is given to a person before a specific microorganism or source of the potential infection is known. It is usually a broad-spectrum antibiotic and the treatment may change if the microorganism or source is confirmed.

Further Reading

1   National Collaborating Centre for Cancer. *Neutropenic sepsis: Prevention and management of neutropenic sepsis in cancer patients. Full guideline.* Guideline developed for NICE. Cardiff: National Collaborating Centre for Cancer; Sep 2012. Available at: www.nice.org.uk/nicemedia/live/13905/60864/60864.pdf

2   Mort D, Lansdown M, Smith N, Protopapa K, Mason M. *For better, for worse? A review of the care of patients who died within 30 days of receiving systemic anti-cancer therapy.* London: National Confidential Enquiry into Patient Outcome and Death (NCEPOD); Nov 2008. 150pp.

3   Freifeld AG, Bow EJ, Sepkowitz KA, *et al.* Clinical practice guideline for the use of antimicrobial agents in neutropenic patients with cancer: 2010 update by the Infectious Diseases Society of America. *Clin Infect Dis* 2011; **52**(4): e56–e93.

4   Sipsas NV, Bodey GP, Kontoyiannis DP. Perspectives for the management of febrile neutropenic patients with cancer in the 21st century. *Cancer* 2005; 103(6): 1103–13.

5   Gafter-Gvili A, Fraser A, Paul M, Vidal L, *et al.* Antibiotic prophylaxis for bacterial infections in afebrile neutropenic patients following chemotherapy. *Cochrane Database Syst Rev* 2012; **1**: CD004386.

6   Cooper K, Madan J, Whyte S, Stevenson M, Akehurst R. Granulocyte colony-stimulating factors for febrile neutropenia prophylaxis following chemotherapy: systematic review and meta-analysis. *BMC Cancer* 2011; **11**(1):404.

7   Aapro MS, Bohlius J, Cameron DA, *et al.* 2010 update of EORTC guidelines for the use of granulocyte-colony stimulating factor to reduce the incidence of chemotherapy-induced febrile neutropenia in adult patients with lymphoproliferative disorders and solid tumours. *Eur J Cancer* 2011; **47**(1): 8–32.

8   Crawford J, Allen J, Armitage J, *et al.* Myeloid growth factors. *J Natl Compr Canc Netw* 2011; **9**(8): 914–32.

9   National Cancer Peer Review–National Cancer Action Team. Acute Oncology Measures. London: National Cancer Peer Review, National Cancer Action Team; 7 Apr 2013. Available at: www.cquins.nhs.uk/?menu=resources

10 Klastersky J, Paesmans M, Edward EB, *et al.* The Multinational Association for Supportive Care in Cancer Risk Index: A multinational scoring system for identifying low risk febrile neutropenic cancer patients. *J Clin Oncol* 2000; **18**(16): 3038–51.

11 Innes H, Lim S, Hall A, Chan S, Bhalla N, Marshall E. Management of febrile neutropenia in solid tumours and lymphomas using the Multinational Association for Supportive Care in Cancer (MASCC) risk index: feasibility and safety in routine clinical practice. *Support Care Cancer* 2008; **16**(5): 485–91.

12 National Chemotherapy Advisory Group. *Chemotherapy Services in England: Ensuring quality and safety.* London: Department of Health; 21 Aug 2009. 70pp.

13 Surviving Sepsis Campaign [Internet]. Bundles. Mount Prospect, Ill.: Society of Critical Care Medicine; c.2001–13. Available from: www.survivingsepsis.org/Bundles/Pages/default.aspx

13 Tumour Lysis Syndrome

Christopher Parrish, Gordon Cook

Case History

A 33-year-old man with newly diagnosed aggressive non-Hodgkin lymphoma is admitted to receive his first cycle of chemotherapy. The patient has no significant medical history and takes no prescribed medicines. His father has glucose-6-phosphate dehydrogenase deficiency.

How may the risk of tumour lysis syndrome be gauged?

What prophylactic therapies are available? Which should the patient receive?

What are the complications of tumour lysis syndrome and how should this patient be monitored?

Background

Tumour lysis syndrome (TLS) is a potentially lethal clinicopathological syndrome caused by rapid lysis of malignant cells. The consequent metabolic derangements give rise to a spectrum of symptoms, which are listed in Table 13.1. TLS may be present prior to treatment, due to high cell turnover, but more usually occurs 12–72 hours after initiation of therapy.

Table 13.1 Clinicopathological features of tumour lysis syndrome (TLS)

Metabolic derangements following tumour breakdown	Spectrum of symptoms associated with TLS
Hyperuricaemia	Lethargy
Hyperkalaemia	Nausea
Hyperphosphataemia	Vomiting
Hypocalcaemia	Fluid overload
Uraemia	Cardiac arrhythmias
	Muscle cramps
	Tetany
	Seizures
	Syncope
	Sudden death

How may the risk of tumour lysis syndrome be gauged?

Factors influencing the risk of TLS may be grouped into disease, patient and treatment factors. Table 13.2 gives a guide to risk assessment for some more common situations in adult oncology, although each patient requires a personalized assessment of risk.

Table 13.2 Evaluation of risk and prophylaxis of tumour lysis syndrome. Adapted from (1).

	Risk Factors	Prophylaxis suggestions
Low risk	• AML with WBC <25×10⁹/l and LDH <2×ULN • CML • HL • MM • NHL, indolent • NHL, intermediate grade with LDH <2×ULN • Most solid tumours	Monitoring Hydration [+-]Allopurinol
Intermediate risk	• ALL with WBC <100×10⁹/l and LDH <2×ULN • AML with WBC 25–100×10⁹/l or WBC <25 and LDH ≥2×ULN • BL stage I/II and LDH <2×ULN • CLL with WBC >50×10⁹/l or treated with fludarabine or rituximab • NHL, intermediate grade with LDH ≥2xULN • LL stage I/II and LDH <2×ULN • Chemosensitive solid tumours (e.g. neuroblastoma, germ cell tumours, SCLC), or those with bulky or advanced stage disease	Monitoring Hydration Allopurinol
High risk	• ALL with WBC ≥100 and/or LDH >2×ULN • AML with WBC ≥100×10⁹/l • BL stage III/IV and/or LDH >2×ULN • IRD with renal dysfunction or involvement • IRD with uric acid, potassium and/or phosphate >ULN • LL stage III/IV and or LDH >2×ULN	Monitoring Hydration Rasburicase

ALL, acute lymphoblastic leukaemia; AML, acute myeloid leukaemia; BL, Burkitt lymphoma; CLL, chronic lymphocytic leukaemia; CML, chronic myeloid leukaemia; HL, Hodgkin lymphoma; IRD, intermediate-risk disease; LDH, lactate dehydrogenase; LL, lymphoblastic lymphoma; MM, multiple myeloma; NHL, non-Hodgkin lymphoma; SCLC, small-cell lung cancer; ULN, upper limit of normal range; WBC, white blood cell count.

Disease factors

Neoplasms that are either highly proliferative or highly sensitive to cytotoxic therapy (there is considerable overlap between these two groups) present a particularly high risk of TLS. High-grade non-Hodgkin lymphoma (in particular Burkitt lymphoma), acute lymphoblastic leukaemia and chemosensitive solid tumours (e.g. neuroblastoma, germ-cell tumours and small-cell lung cancer) are the cancers primarily associated with TLS, although attempts at a more sophisticated classification have been made.[1] A large burden of disease further increases the risk; its assessment varies between malignancies but typically encompasses clinical and radiological examination, as well as blood and bone marrow examination for haematological malignancies. Serum lactate dehydrogenase is a useful surrogate marker of disease burden. Bulky tumours, adenopathy and organomegaly obviously represent high-volume disease, but high circulating white cell counts ($>100\times10^9$/l) in acute leukaemia, chronic myeloid leukaemia in blast crisis and high-count chronic lymphocytic leukaemia should also be considered high risk. Histologically high-grade disease and immunohistological and molecular markers of highly proliferative disease (e.g. high Ki-67 antigen staining) also indicate increased risk of TLS.

Patient factors
Any coincident medical condition that impairs the patient's ability to clear metabolites of lysed malignant cells will increase the risk of TLS. Pre-existing renal dysfunction, urinary tract obstruction by tumour, intravascular volume depletion and coincident sepsis are common complications in the setting of malignancy.

Treatment factors
More potent therapies, resulting in more marked cytotoxicity, necessarily increase the risk of TLS. For example, addition of the anti-CD20 monoclonal antibody rituximab to conventional alkylating agent-based therapies considerably increases the risk of TLS when treating B-cell lymphomas. The first cycle of therapy may be attenuated to ameliorate this hazard. It should be noted that introduction of novel, more potent, therapies may increase the risk of TLS for a given disease.

What prophylactic therapies are available? Which should the patient receive?
Prophylaxis against TLS should be considered for all patients commencing chemotherapy; the modalities used will depend on the level of risk. Where possible, cytotoxic therapy should be delayed until adequate prophylaxis has been given.

Hydration
In the absence of acute renal dysfunction, vigorous hydration and diuresis improves intravascular volume, renal blood flow, glomerular filtration and urinary excretion of uric acid and phosphate, and is a mainstay of therapy. Potassium, calcium and phosphate should not be added to initial intravenous fluids. In high-risk situations, fluid therapy to maintain urine output ≥100 ml/m^2/h is often recommended.[2] If urine output remains suboptimal, and once obstructive nephropathy and hypovolaemia have been excluded, diuretics such as mannitol or furosemide may be considered. Urinary alkalinization, traditionally recommended to augment urate excretion, is no longer routinely employed due to its propensity to induce renal crystallization of xanthine and hypoxanthine when used concomitantly with allopurinol.

Allopurinol and rasburicase
The xanthine oxidase inhibitor allopurinol prevents conversion of hypoxanthine and xanthine to uric acid; the resultant oxypurine accumulation is renally excreted. There are, however, a number of considerations with the use of this agent. Firstly, allopurinol only prevents the formation of new uric acid, and has no impact on existing levels. Secondly,

doses of azathioprine, 6-mercaptopurine, thioguanine and other drugs metabolized by xanthine oxidase must be reduced. In addition, renally excreted oxypurines may crystallize and cause obstructive nephropathy.

A newer agent, rasburicase (recombinant urate oxidase, an enzyme lacking in humans), catalyses the conversion of uric acid to allantoin, which is far more soluble in urine. This has the advantage of clearing existing uric acid in addition to preventing further accumulation. The drug is expensive, although there is evidence that a single dose may suffice.[3]

The choice between the two agents hinges on assessing the risk of TLS on an individual basis: rasburicase should be considered for high-risk situations, e.g. initial chemotherapy for Burkitt lymphoma. It should be noted that both protect only against hyperuricaemia – the other biochemical complications of TLS are unaffected. With reference to the case history, glucose-6-phosphate dehydrogenase deficiency (G6PDd) is a contraindication to rasburicase, which may precipitate haemolysis in this condition. However, since G6PDd is X-linked recessive the patient has only the population background risk of having the disorder – it may be appropriate to screen high-risk populations prior to rasburicase therapy.

What are the complications of tumour lysis syndrome and how should they be managed?

Complications of TLS may precede initiation of therapy in highly proliferative malignancies, but more usually occur 12–72 hours afterwards. Patients should be monitored closely for deterioration in renal function and serum levels of urate, phosphate, potassium and calcium.

Hyperphosphataemia, which is typically asymptomatic unless severe, should generally be treated once phosphorus levels exceed 2.1 mmol/l. Initial measures are avoidance of phosphate in intravenous fluids and diet, and oral phosphate-binding resins (e.g. aluminium hydroxide). Where severe, renal replacement therapy may be required, with haemodialysis being the modality of choice.[4]

Hypocalcaemia requires careful management since intravenous supplementation of calcium may result in precipitation of calcium phosphate, leading to metastatic calcification; this is of grave concern as it gives rise to intrarenal calcification, nephrocalcinosis, nephrolithiasis and obstructive uropathy.[5] For this reason, calcium gluconate 50–100 mg/kg IV should be given, cautiously, only if hypocalcaemia is symptomatic.

Asymptomatic hyperkalaemia requires avoidance of oral and IV potassium, cessation of exacerbating drugs, electrocardiographic monitoring and calcium-free oral exchange resins (e.g. sodium polystyrene sulphonate). If hyperkalaemia is symptomatic, insulin/dextrose infusion, nebulized salbutamol (unlicensed indication in EU and USA) and/or IV calcium gluconate will be required; the latter may increase the risk of metastatic calcification as already discussed. Resistant hyperkalaemia may require dialysis.

Hyperuricaemia is best prevented through appropriate use of prophylactic agents as discussed above. However, rasburicase also has activity in established TLS and should be considered in this setting.[6,7]

Uraemia and acute renal dysfunction may be multifactorial during TLS, with obstructive nephropathy due to uric acid crystals, intrarenal calcification, nephrocalcinosis and nephrolithiasis adding to the existing problems of renal tumour infiltration, obstructive uropathy due to malignant masses, nephrotoxic drugs and intravascular volume depletion. Careful management of the complications of TLS as described above is critically important, as is monitoring of fluid balance, reducing doses of renally excreted medicines, and management of hypertension. Nevertheless, acute renal dysfunction, like the electrolyte disturbances discussed above, may necessitate a period of renal replacement therapy, and a nephrologist should be involved early.

Conclusions

TLS is a potentially life-threatening complication of aggressive malignancies and their associated treatments, with a range of clinicopathological manifestations. The risk of TLS is dictated by disease, patient and treatment factors, and requires assessment on an individual patient basis before initiation of treatment. Prophylactic therapy with fluids, allopurinol and rasburicase can reduce the risk of TLS and its complications. However, patients must be monitored closely for metabolic derangements, which should be corrected, and early multidisciplinary input is often needed. Given the markedly adverse prognosis associated with the condition, early consideration of TLS and assessment of risk are crucial steps in the safe initiation of anticancer therapy.

Further reading

1   Cairo MS, Coiffier B, Reiter A, Younes A; TLS Expert Panel. Recommendations for the evaluation of risk and prophylaxis of tumour lysis syndrome (TLS) in adults and children with malignant diseases: an expert TLS panel consensus. *Br J Haematol* 2010; **149**: 578–86.

2   Abu-Alfa AK, Younes A. Tumor lysis syndrome and acute kidney injury: evaluation, prevention, and management. *Am J Kidney Dis* 2010; **55**: S1–S13.

3   Vadhan-Raj S, Fayad LE, Fanale MA, *et al.* A randomized trial of a single-dose rasburicase versus five-daily doses in patients at risk for tumor lysis syndrome. *Ann Oncol* 2012; **23**: 1640–45.

4   Jones DP, MahmoudH, Chesney RW. Tumor lysis syndrome: pathogenesis and management. *Pediatr Nephrol* 1995; **9**: 206–12.

5   Cairo MS, Bishop M. Tumour lysis syndrome: new therapeutic strategies and classification. *Br J Haematol* 2004; **127**: 3–11.

6   Pui CH, Mahmoud HH, Wiley JM, *et al.* Recombinant urate oxidase for the prophylaxis or treatment of hyperuricemia in patients with leukemia or lymphoma. *J Clin Oncol* 2001; **19**: 697–704.

7   Coiffier B, Mounier N, Bologna S, *et al.* Efficacy and safety of rasburicase (recombinant urate oxidase) for the prevention and treatment of hyperuricemia during induction chemotherapy of aggressive non-Hodgkin's lymphoma: results of the GRAAL1 (Groupe d'Etude des Lymphomes de l'Adulte Trial on Rasburicase Activity in Adult Lymphoma) study. *J Clin Oncol* 2003; **21**: 4402–6.

PROBLEM

14 Antiangiogenic Therapy

Gordon Urquhart, Fiona Collinson

Case History

A 65-year-old patient with metastatic clear-cell carcinoma of the kidney is waiting to be seen in the outpatient clinic. The patient is attending for a drug toxicity review, having started sunitinib three weeks ago.

During treatment the patient has experienced intermittent nose bleeds, indigestion, and soreness to his hands and feet. His wife has noticed a yellow tinge to his skin and swelling of his eyelids. The clinic nurse is concerned by his elevated blood pressure recordings.

What class of drug is sunitinib, and what other angiogenic agents exist in clinical use?

What are the side-effects of inhibiting angiogenesis?

How should this patient be managed with regards to toxicity from antiangiogenic therapy?

Background

What class of drug is sunitinib?

Sunitinib, delivered orally, inhibits multiple receptor tyrosine kinases (RTKs) that are involved in angiogenesis, tumour growth and metastatic progression of cancer.[1-4] The antiangiogenic effect results from inhibition of vascular endothelial growth factor receptors (VEGFR) VEGFR1, VEGFR2 and VEGFR3.[1,2] In addition, sunitinib also inhibits platelet-derived growth factor receptors (PDGFR) PDGFRA and PDGFRB, stem cell growth factor receptor (KIT), fms-related tyrosine kinase 3 (FLT3), colony-stimulating factor 1 receptor (CSF1R), and the glial cell line-derived neurotrophic factor receptor (RET).[1,2,4]

Are there other drugs in clinical use that target angiogenesis?

There are now a number of therapeutic agents available for use in clinical practice that target angiogenesis (the formation of new blood vessels) to slow tumour growth and metastasis. Some of the common drugs are listed in Table 14.1.

The angiogenesis-related signalling pathways are important to physiological response and homeostasis in many tissues and organs. They play important roles in haematopoiesis, myelopoiesis, endothelial cell survival, tissue growth and wound healing.[1,2] Accordingly, the blockage of these pathways by inhibitors has produced a wide range of toxicities, which are determined by the sites of action of the individual drugs (Table 14.2).

Table 14.1 Drugs targeting angiogenesis			
Drug Name	Molecular Targets*	Drug Type	Clinical Indication
Axitinib	VEGFR1 VEGFR2 VEGFR3 PDGFR KIT	Small molecule TKI	Renal
Bevacizumab	VEGFR	Monoclonal antibody	Breast Colorectal Lung Ovarian
Pazopanib	VEGFR1 VEGFR2 VEGFR3	Small molecule TKI	Renal Soft tissue sarcoma
Sorafenib	VEGFR2 VEGFR3 VEGFR3 PDGFR RAF1 KIT FLT3	Small molecule TKI	Hepatocellular Renal Glioblastoma multiforme
Sunitinib	VEGFR1 VEGFR2 PDGFR KIT FLT3 RET	Small molecule TKI	Renal Gastrointestinal stromal tumour

*See earlier description of molecular targets in main text. TKI, tyrosine kinase inhibitor.

What are the likely side-effects of inhibiting angiogenesis?

Hair
Discoloration or depigmentation of hair has been commonly observed. With sunitinib this can result in a striped hair colour, as the discoloration of hair closely follows the treatment schedule of four weeks of treatment followed by two weeks of rest.

Eyes
Eyelid oedema is commonly observed and in the absence of significant proteinuria is generally without sequelae.

Mouth
Oral mucositis and taste alteration are commonly reported and treated with typical mouth care regimes.

Thyroid

VEGF inhibition can result in disturbed thyroid cell function with an increase in thyroid-stimulating hormone levels, a decrease in the levels of circulating thyroid hormones and symptoms consistent with hypothyroidism. This is most commonly in patients treated with sunitinib (10%–36%).[1,3,4] It is less common with sorafenib, and is not evident with bevacizumab.

Skin

Skin discoloration with a yellow tinge, due to a colourant in the active substance, is a common (30%) adverse reaction in patients treated with sunitinib.[4] Other common toxicities found with most agents include: dryness, thickness or cracking of the skin; blistering; palmar-plantar erythrodysaesthesia; and an acne form rash, typically with the tyrosine kinase inhibitors. Dermatological toxicities can be managed with topical therapies for symptomatic relief, treatment interruption or dose reduction.

Cardiovascular

Hypertension is a common toxicity associated with all inhibitors of angiogenesis. Inhibition of VEGF can cause a decrease in the release of known vasodilators (nitric oxide and prostacyclin) from endothelial cells, with a consequent rise in blood pressure.[1,2,5] Additionally, VEGF inhibition disturbs baroreceptor response and increases the activity of endothelin, and both effects have been proposed as mechanisms for the development of hypertension.[1,2] Risk factors for developing hypertension during treatment include pre-existing hypertension as well as a diagnosis of metastatic renal cell carcinoma. The effect of VEGF inhibition on blood pressure appears to be dose dependent.[2,5] Optimization of hypertensive medication using a variety of agents, including diuretics, β-blockers, angiotensin-converting enzyme inhibitors and calcium channel blockers, has been used to achieve blood pressure control in line with current standards.

Reduced left ventricular ejection fraction and congestive heart failure (CHF) have been reported with both bevacizumab and sunitinib.[6,7] In a meta-analysis evaluating the incidence of cardiac toxicity with sunitinib, high-grade (≥grade 3) CHF was reported in 1.5% of patients. Congestive heart failure of any grade was identified in 4.15% of patients treated with sunitinib.[7] In patients with imatinib-refractory gastrointestinal stromal tumour (GIST) treated with sunitinib rates of CHF up to 8% were reported.[6] In metastatic breast cancer patients pre-treated with anthracycline, CHF has been reported in 2% of patients on bevacizumab therapy.[1,2]

Gastrointestinal

The risk of gastrointestinal perforation and fistula formation is increased with the use of VEGF inhibitors. In metastatic colorectal cancer the risk of perforation increased from 0% in a chemotherapy-only group to 1.5% in the bevacizumab and chemotherapy treatment arm.[5] Although perforation appears most often within the tumour area, its occurrence at sites of inflammation or ulceration has also been reported. Sunitinib and sorafenib have less commonly been associated with gastrointestinal perforation.

The mucosal inflammation induced by treatment can result in dyspepsia, nausea, vomiting and diarrhoea, and these side effects are most commonly reported as Common Terminology Criteria for Adverse Events (CTCAE) grades 1 or 2. Concomitant medications are usually successful when given to help relieve these toxicities.

Table 14.2 Side-effects of antiangiogenic drugs

Organ	Toxicity
Hair	Depigmentation
Eyes	Eyelid oedema
Mouth	Loss of taste
	Mucositis
Thyroid	Hypothyroidism
Skin	Discoloration
	Palmar-plantar erythrodysaesthesia
	Rash
Cardiovascular	Hypertension
	Cardiac failure
Gastrointestinal	Diarrhoea
	Dyspepsia
	Fistula
	Nausea
	Perforation
	Stomatitis
Haematological	Anaemia
	Haemorrhage
	Leukopenia
	Neutropenia
	Thrombocytopenia
	Thromboembolic events
Renal	Proteinuria

Wound healing is reliant upon angiogenesis. Surgery on patients with colorectal cancer during bevacizumab plus chemotherapy resulted in increased problems with wound healing compared to treatment with chemotherapy alone. Most clinical trials using antiangiogenic treatments require a minimum of 14–28 days from surgery (dependent on the drug used) before commencing such treatments.[5]

Haematological and thrombotic events
The risk of both spontaneous mucosal and tumour bleeding is increased with treatment. Although mild epistaxis is the most common presentation, clinical trials have reported severe and life-threatening bleeding episodes. Bevacizumab is now contraindicated in squamous non-small-cell lung carcinomas as a consequence of this increased bleeding risk.

In clinical trials, treatment with bevacizumab was associated with an increased risk of arterial thromboembolic events, with 3.8% in the bevacizumab treatment groups compared to 1.7% in the control groups.[1,2,5] Cerebrovascular accidents were reported in up to 2.3% of patients treated with bevacizumab in combination with chemotherapy, compared to 0.5% of patients treated with chemotherapy alone.[5] Treatment-related venous thromboembolic events were reported in approximately 1% of patients with solid tumours who received sunitinib on clinical trials, including those treated for GIST and metastatic renal cell carcinoma (MRCC).[1,2] Sunitinib is known to induce neutropenia (grade 3 = 8%–11%) and thrombocytopenia (grade 3 = 4%–8%), as is sorafenib (grade 3 neutropenia = 5%; grade 3 thrombocytopenia = 1%).[1-3] However, bevacizumab alone does not appear to induce myelosuppression.

Renal
Although asymptomatic and mild proteinuria is common with bevacizumab, it is far less common with the small-molecule tyrosine kinase inhibitors. It rarely progresses to nephrotic syndrome (<0.5%) and usually resolves on withdrawal of the medication.

How should this patient be managed?
The patient in this case was seen by a consultant with experience in the management of patients with antiangiogenic therapy and a specialist nurse in the renal clinic. The severity of the symptoms and the elevation of blood pressure were deemed to represent a significant risk to the patient and his sunitinib dose was stopped. Three weeks later the patient re-started treatment at 75% of the initial dose and he tolerated his second cycle of treatment well. His blood pressure was monitored frequently using a home blood pressure monitor and he was seen at two-week intervals in the clinic, where minor adjustments in his antihypertensive treatment were necessary. The patient was able to tolerate four further cycles of sunitinib and achieved a good partial response to therapy lasting over a year.

Conclusion

The inhibitors of angiogenesis represent an important class of cancer therapy in an increasing number of tumour sites. The side-effect profiles are wide ranging, and managing this toxicity will be an important aspect of acute oncology.

Further reading

1   Chen HX, Cleck JN. Adverse effects of anticancer agents that target the VEGF pathway. *Nat Rev Clin Oncol* 2009; **6**: 465–77.

2   Verheaul HMW, Pinedo HM. Possible molecular mechanisms involved in the toxicity of angiogenesis inhibition. *Nat Rev Cancer* 2007; **7**: 475–85.

3   Gore ME, Szczylik C, Porta C, *et al.* Safety and efficacy of sunitnib for metastatic renal-cell carcinoma: an expanded-access trial. *Lancet* 2009; **10**: 757–63.

4   Motzer RJ, Hutson TE, Tomczak, *et al.* Sunitinib versus interferon alfa in metastatic renal-cell carcinoma. *N Engl J Med* 2007; **356**(2): 115–24.[AQ1]

5   Shih T, Lindley C. Bevacizumab: an angiogenesis inhibitor for the treatment of solid malignancies. *Clin Ther* 2006; **28**(11): 1779–802.

6   Chu TF, Rupnick MA, Kerkela R, *et al.* Cardiotoxicity associated with tyrosine kinase inhibitor sunitinib. *Lancet* 2007; **370**: 2011–9.

7   Richards CJ, Je Y, Schutz FA, *et al.* Incidence and risk of congestive heart failure in patients with renal and nonrenal cell carcinoma treated with sunitinib. *J Clin Oncol* 2011; **29**(25): 3450–6.

15 Cardiac Toxicity

Pankaj Punia, Chris Plummer

Case History

A 67-year-old woman presented with a 1.9 cm nodule in her left breast. Biopsy revealed a grade 3 infiltrating ductal cancer which was ER-negative, PR-negative and HER2-positive. A lumpectomy with sentinel node dissection was performed. Two out of four nodes were found to be positive for metastasis. She underwent complete axillary node clearance. All other nodes were clear of cancer.

Her past history included hypertension controlled with ramipril, and diet-controlled diabetes. She was an ex-smoker with a 20 pack-year smoking history. Her ECG showed sinus rhythm and was within normal limits. Her routine bloods tests were all normal.

The patient was keen to try any treatment option to reduce her risk of recurrence. A plan was made to start anthracycline-based chemotherapy followed by docetaxel and then trastuzumab for one year.

What are the patient's risk factors for cardiac toxicity with anthracycline and trastuzumab?

What is the mechanism of cardiac toxicity?

What is current clinical evidence available to support this?

How would you manage and follow up this patient?

Are there any other cytotoxic drugs with potential to cause cardiac toxicity? What are common cardiotoxicities associated with these agents?

Background

What are the patient's risk factors for cardiac toxicity with anthracycline and trastuzumab?

A number of risk factors have been identified for increased likelihood of cardiac toxicity with anthracyclines and trastuzumab.

Anthracycline

The strongest predictor of cardiac toxicity is cumulative dose. Although there is a wide range of individual susceptibilities, doses above 300 mg/m^2 of doxorubicin or 900 mg/m^2 of epirubicin are associated with a higher incidence of heart failure events.[1-3] Dose schedule, reflecting peak plasma concentration, is a significant risk modifier, with bolus administration posing a higher risk than continuous infusion.[3] There is also evidence that concurrent administration of other agents which affect heart function (e.g. trastuzumab) increases toxicity, and that liposomal formulations are less toxic.[4,5] Patient risk factors include age, with those >65 years having a higher risk of events at a given dose.[6] There is equivocal evidence for other risk factors, including chest radiotherapy and pre-existing cardiovascular disease (coronary artery disease, hypertension, peripheral vascular disease and diabetes).[7,8]

Trastuzumab

Trastuzumab is a monoclonal antibody directed against HER2. The effect of this agent on heart function does not appear to be related to peak concentration or cumulative dose. As noted above, prior or especially concurrent exposure to anthracycline greatly increases the risk of cardiac toxicity.[9] In contrast, concurrent radiation therapy does not appear to increase that risk.[10] Other factors associated with an increased risk of cardiac events with trastuzumab-containing regimens include pre-existing cardiac dysfunction, and hypertension requiring the use of antihypertensive medication.[11]

What is the mechanism of cardiac toxicity?

Anthracyclines

Cardiac toxicity is a well-known adverse effect of anthracyclines, but its underlying mechanism remains incompletely understood. Cardiac damage has been attributed to the production of toxic reactive oxygen species (free radicals) and a subsequent increase in oxidative stress, which can lead to irreversible damage as myocytes are replaced by fibrous tissue.[7] Myocardial iron accumulation may also play a direct role in anthracycline cardiac toxicity.

Trastuzumab

Epidermal growth factor signalling involving HER2 has been shown to be important in the normal heart, and this suggests that trastuzumab's cardiotoxic effects are directly related to HER2 blockade. Trastuzumab blocks HER2-mediated signalling and thus interferes with the heart's ability to respond to stress.[12]

Anthracycline-associated cardiac dysfunction is dose-related and appears to cause permanent myocardial damage, whereas trastuzumab-associated cardiac dysfunction is typically reversible, is not dose-related and does not appear to produce the typical morphological changes associated with anthracycline.[13]

What is current clinical evidence available to support this?

Anthracycline

Anthracycline-based adjuvant breast cancer treatment is associated with a 10% absolute increase in heart failure events at 10 years' follow-up.[14]

Trastuzumab

In the North Central Cancer Treatment Group (NCCTG) N9831 trial, 2992 patients received doxorubicin plus cyclophosphamide (AC) for adjuvant breast cancer treatment. During treatment with AC, 5% of patients had falls in left ventricular ejection fraction (LVEF) such that they did not receive trastuzumab. Of those receiving subsequent paclitaxel alone, 0.3% experienced a heart failure event or cardiac death, compared to 2.8% of those receiving sequential paclitaxel then trastuzumab, and 3.3% of those receiving paclitaxel and trastuzumab concurrently.[11,15]

In the National Surgical Adjuvant Breast and Bowel Project (NSABP) B-31 trial, following AC chemotherapy and the demonstration of normal cardiac function, 814 patients were randomized to paclitaxel alone, and 850 to paclitaxel and trastuzumab. Of the group receiving paclitaxel alone, 0.8% had a heart failure event during three-year follow-up, versus 4.1% in the paclitaxel and trastuzumab group.[16]

The Herceptin Adjuvant (HERA) trial compared one year of treatment with trastuzumab with observation after surgery, radiotherapy and neoadjuvant or adjuvant chemotherapy in patients with HER2-positive early breast cancer and adequate cardiac function. After a two-year follow-up, the incidence of severe heart failure (NYHA class III or IV) was 0.6% in the trastuzumab arm and 0% in the observation arm. There were no cardiac deaths in the trastuzumab arm compared to one (0.1%) in the observation arm.[17]

How would you manage and follow up this patient?

When treatment is planned for patients in the adjuvant or metastatic setting, the patient's risk for anthracycline and trastuzumab-related cardiac toxicity should be carefully assessed and weighed against the benefits of such treatment.

Trastuzumab therapy should be started after LVEF has been shown to be within the normal range in both the adjuvant and metastatic settings.[16] To ensure the early identification of cardiac dysfunction, LVEF assessments should be repeated every three months during trastuzumab treatment. National Institute for Health and Care Excellence (NICE) guidance published in 2006 states that if the LVEF drops by 10% (ejection fraction) or more from baseline and to below 50% then trastuzumab treatment should be suspended.[18] More recent guidance recommends starting an ACE inhibitor if there is a ≥10% fall in LVEF to below the lower limit of normal, but continuing trastuzumab in asymptomatic patients unless the LVEF is ≤40%. A decision to resume trastuzumab therapy after recovery of LVEF should be based on a further cardiac assessment and an informed discussion of the risk and benefits between the individual patient and their clinician. Trastuzumab-related cardiac toxicity usually responds to standard medical treatment for heart failure and the discontinuation of trastuzumab in most cases, but if there is any doubt specialist cardiology opinion should be sought early.

Dexrazoxane is an EDTA-like chelator that was shown to have efficacy in reducing the risk of anthracycline-related cardiac toxicity in a meta-analysis of six randomized trials.[3] Its use has been limited since the publication of two trials suggesting an increased risk of secondary malignancy.[20]

Are there any other cytotoxic drugs with potential to cause cardiac toxicity? What are common cardiotoxicities associated with these agents?

Other chemotherapeutic agents associated with significant risk of cardiac adverse effects include alkylating agents, fluorouracil, paclitaxel and vinca alkaloids. Cardiovascular side-effects are also associated with the use of targeted therapies, such as monoclonal antibodies and tyrosine kinase inhibitors.[21]

Cardiac events may include mild blood pressure changes, thrombosis, ECG changes, arrhythmias, myocarditis, pericarditis, myocardial infarction, cardiomyopathy and left ventricular failure. These may occur within days, weeks or months after treatment. Risks for cardiotoxicity should be recognized before therapy is initiated and action should be taken to modify them if necessary. Monitoring and treatment for cardiac events will usually depend on the signs and symptoms anticipated and exhibited.

Table 15.1	Main cardiotoxicity of chemotherapeutic agents	
Cardiotoxic side effect	**Chemotherapeutic agents associated**
Hypertension	Monoclonal antibodies e.g. bevacizumab
	Tyrosinase kinase inhibitors e.g. sunitinib, pazopanib, sorafenib
Heart failure	Anthracyclines, e.g. epirubicin, doxorubicin
	HER2 receptor inhibitors, e.g. trastuzumab, lapatinib
Acute coronary syndrome	Fluorouracil, e.g. 5-fluorouracil, capecitabine
	Vinca alkaloids, e.g. vincristine, vinorelbine
Arrhythmias	Platinum agents, e.g. cisplatin, carboplatin
	Alkylating agents, e.g. cyclophosphamide , ifosfamide, melphalan

Conclusion

This patient has high-risk breast cancer. She will get maximum benefit with a combination of anthracycline and trastuzumab-based adjuvant chemotherapy. There are several risk factors which increase the patient's risk of cardiotoxicity. She will require close cardiac monitoring and assessment during treatment.

Further reading

1   Von Hoff DD, Layard MW, Basa P. Risk factors for doxorubicin-induced congestive heart failure. *Ann Intern Med* 1979; **91**(5): 710–7.

2   Buzdar AU, Marcus C, Smith TL, Blumenschein GR. Early and delayed clinical cardiotoxicity of doxorubicin. *Cancer* 1985; **55**(12): 2761–5.

3   Smith LA, Cornelius VR, Plummer CJ, *et al*. Cardiotoxicity of anthracycline agents for the treatment of cancer: systematic review and meta-analysis of randomised controlled trials. *BMC Cancer* 2010; **10**: 337.

4   Seidman A, Hudis C, Pierri MK, *et al*. Cardiac dysfunction in the trastuzumab clinical trials experience. *J Clin Oncol* 2002; **20**(5): 1215–21.

5   Airoldi M, Amadori D, Barni S, *et al*. Clinical activity and cardiac tolerability of non-pegylated liposomal doxorubicin in breast cancer: a synthetic review. *Tumori* 2011; **97**(6): 690–2.

6   Swain SM, Whaley FS, Ewer MS. Congestive heart failure in patients treated with doxorubicin: a retrospective analysis of three trials. *Cancer* 2003; **97**(11): 2869–79.

7   Singal PK, Deally CM, Weinberg LE. Subcellular effects of adriamycin in the heart: a concise review. *J Mol Cell Cardiol* 1987; **19**(8): 817–28.

8   Hershman DL, McBride RB, Eisenberger A, Tsai WY, Grann VR, Jacobson JS. Doxorubicin, cardiac risk factors, and cardiac toxicity in elderly patients with diffuse B-cell non-Hodgkin's lymphoma. *J Clin Oncol* 2008; **26**(19): 3159–65.

9   Russell SD, Blackwell KL, Lawrence J, *et al.* Independent adjudication of symptomatic heart failure with the use of doxorubicin and cyclophosphamide followed by trastuzumab adjuvant therapy: a combined review of cardiac data from the National Surgical Adjuvant breast and Bowel Project B-31 and the North Central Cancer Treatment Group N9831 clinical trials. *J Clin Oncol* 2010; **28**(21): 3416–21.

10 Halyard MY, Pisansky TM, Dueck AC, *et al.* Radiotherapy and adjuvant trastuzumab in operable breast cancer: tolerability and adverse event data from the NCCTG Phase III Trial N9831. *J Clin Oncol* 2009; **27**(16): 2638–44.

11 Perez EA, Suman VJ, Davidson NE, *et al.* Cardiac safety analysis of doxorubicin and cyclophosphamide followed by paclitaxel with or without trastuzumab in the North Central Cancer Treatment Group N9831 adjuvant breast cancer trial. *J Clin Oncol* 2008; **26**(8): 1231–8.

12 Chien KR. Herceptin and the heart – a molecular modifier of cardiac failure. *N Engl J Med* 2006; **354**(8): 789–90.

13 Ewer MS, Lippman SM. Type II chemotherapy-related cardiac dysfunction: time to recognize a new entity. *J Clin Oncol* 2005; **23**(13): 2900–2.

14 Pinder MC, Duan Z, Goodwin JS, Hortobagyi GN, Giordano SH. Congestive heart failure in older women treated with adjuvant anthracycline chemotherapy for breast cancer. *J Clin Oncol* 2007; **25**(25): 3808–15.

15 Perez EA, Romond EH, Suman VJ, *et al.* Four-year follow-up of trastuzumab plus adjuvant chemotherapy for operable human epidermal growth factor receptor 2-positive breast cancer: joint analysis of data from NCCTG N9831 and NSABP B-31. *J Clin Oncol* 2011; **29**(25): 3366–73.

16 Tan-Chiu E, Yothers G, Romond E, *et al.* Assessment of cardiac dysfunction in a randomized trial comparing doxorubicin and cyclophosphamide followed by paclitaxel, with or without trastuzumab as adjuvant therapy in node-positive, human epidermal growth factor receptor 2-overexpressing breast cancer: NSABP B-31. *J Clin Oncol* 2005; **23**(31): 7811–9.

17 Smith I, Procter M, Gelber RD, *et al.* 2-year follow-up of trastuzumab after adjuvant chemotherapy in HER2-positive breast cancer: a randomised controlled trial. *Lancet* 2007; **369**(9555): 29–36.

18 Ward S, Pilgrim H, Hind D. Trastuzumab for the treatment of primary breast cancer in HER2-positive women: a single technology appraisal. *Health Technol Assess* 2009; **13** (Suppl 1): 1–6.

19 Jones AL, Barlow M, Barrett-Lee PJ, *et al.* Management of cardiac health in trastuzumab-treated patients with breast cancer: updated United Kingdom National Cancer Research Institute recommendations for monitoring. *Br J Cancer* 2009; **100**(5): 684–92.

20 Salzer WL, Devidas M, Carroll WL, *et al.* Long-term results of the pediatric oncology group studies for childhood acute lymphoblastic leukemia 1984-2001: a report from the children's oncology group. *Leukemia* 2010; **24**(2): 355–70.

21 Albini A, Pennesi G, Donatelli F, Cammarota R, De Flora S, Noonan DM. Cardiotoxicity of anticancer drugs: the need for cardio-oncology and cardio-oncological prevention. *J Natl Cancer Inst* 2010; **102**(1): 14–25.

16 Liver Problems

Luis Daverede, Dan Swinson, Rebecca Jones

Case History

A 42-year-old woman of black African origin born in the Gambia received three cycles of neoadjuvant chemotherapy with epirubicin and cyclophosphamide (EC) for a 3 cm, grade III, node-positive, invasive carcinoma of the right breast.

The patient was known to have chronic hepatitis B infection in the low replicative phase (previously called carrier state). Eight months before commencing chemotherapy, her hepatitis B serology was HBsAg-positive and HBeAg-negative. Her viral load was low (<20 IU/ml) and her alanine transaminase (ALT) was 20 IU/l.

Other past medical history included hypertension, malaria, sickle cell trait, and gallstone disease requiring laparoscopic cholecystectomy.

She had elevated transaminases following her third cycle of chemotherapy, with ALT 412 IU/l (ref. range <40 IU/l); bilirubin, alkaline phosphatase (ALP) and albumin were within the normal range.

What is the differential diagnosis and is it likely to be related to hepatitis B?

What steps would you consider to establish the aetiology of this patient's liver disease?

What is the mechanism of hepatitis B virus (HBV) reactivation during immunosuppressive therapies and how can it be prevented?

What are the principles of management of hepatitis and liver failure?

Could this patient's chemotherapy have caused the elevated ALT and is it safe to be continued?

Background

What is the differential diagnosis and is it likely to be related to hepatitis B?

Differential diagnoses include reactivation of hepatitis B, drug-induced liver injury, or other acute viral hepatitis. Although less likely, disease-related liver replacement, biliary obstruction, ischaemic hepatitis secondary to sequestration of sickle cells, and autoimmune hepatitis are possible causes.

Unfortunately, in this patient prophylactic antivirals for her HBV carrier status were not initiated at the outset of her chemotherapy. Following diagnosis of reactivation she received treatment with tenofovir 245 mg once a day. The HBV DNA levels, having been significantly raised, reduced to <20 IU/ml and the patient's liver function recovered (Table 16.1). She was able to resume her chemotherapy after a five-week delay, but remained under close surveillance by the hepatology team. The standard chemotherapy regimen was modified, with an earlier switch to a taxane and trastuzumab at cycle 4. The patient responded well to the chemotherapy and underwent a mastectomy as originally planned, with clear resection margins.

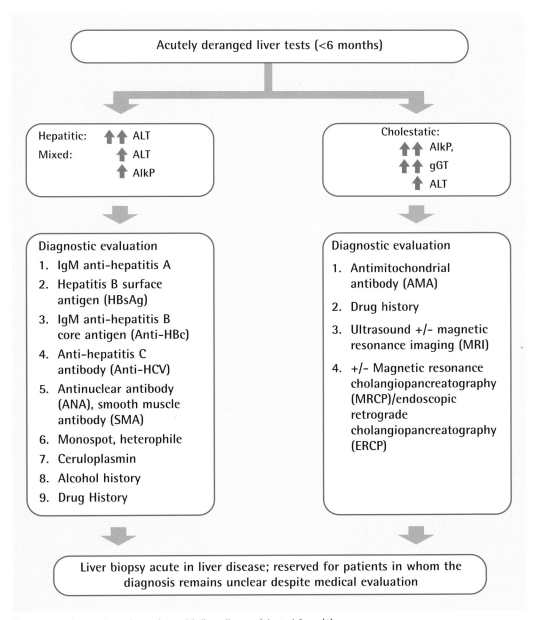

Figure 16.1 Approach to the patient with liver disease. Adapted from (1).

What steps would you consider to establish the aetiology of this patient's liver disease?

It is important to distinguish the pattern of liver disease when establishing a differential diagnosis, usually classified as hepatocellular (or hepatitic), cholestatic or mixed.

The algorithm in Figure 16.1 gives a methodical approach to abnormal liver tests.

In this particular patient, who presents with a hepatitic pattern, the differential diagnosis must include HBV reactivation, other viral hepatitis, drug-induced liver toxicity and metastatic liver lesions. This patient's hepatitis C and hepatitis D serology was negative. Hepatitis A serology should have also been included, as should serological markers for autoimmune disease, e.g. antinuclear antibody and anti-smooth muscle antibody with an immunoglobulin profile.

The hepatitis B viral load was high, confirming the main differential diagnosis, hepatitis B reactivation.

What is the mechanism of hepatitis B virus (HBV) reactivation during immunosuppressive therapies and how can it be prevented?

The World Health Organization estimates that the prevalence of HBV in the UK is 0.3%. Due to immigration from areas of high prevalence, this is likely to increase. Endemic areas include south-east Asia and the Pacific Basin (excluding Japan, Australia, and New Zealand), sub-Saharan Africa, the Amazon Basin, parts of the Middle East, the central Asian Republics, and some countries in Eastern Europe. In countries such as China, Senegal and Thailand, infection rates are very high in infants and continue through early childhood.[2]

HBV persists in the liver even after successful immunological control of the infection and can reactivate during periods of immunosuppression. Reactivations are more common with haematological malignancies and haematopoietic stem cell transplantation (HSCT), but can occur during treatment of solid tumours.[3]

The liver damage in HBV reactivation occurs in two stages: initially there is an enhanced viral replication during immunosuppressive therapy, and then, with restoration of the immune function, a rapid immune-mediated destruction of infected hepatocytes.[3] Reactivation is therefore often seen between cycles of chemotherapy or at the end of a course, and as a result patients remain at risk of hepatitis B reactivation for several months after the end of their cancer treatment.

Lamivudine is a nucleoside analogue that inhibits HBV replication. A meta-analysis of studies using prophylactic lamivudine in hepatitis B-positive cancer patients receiving myelosuppressive chemotherapy showed a significant reduction in all-cause mortality (OR 0.36; 95% CI 0.23–0.56).[4]

Guidelines for the prevention of HBV reactivation during immunosuppressive therapy may be available locally within specialist networks.[5]

Patients should be assessed by a hepatologist or gastroenterologist to determine whether hepatitis B treatment is required, and if not, whether prophylactic therapy to cover the period of reactivation risk is needed. The use of prophylaxis should be implemented according to the patient's individual risk, based on the following:

1. Patient's serology

2. Level of myelosuppression

3. HBV DNA levels.

Time of test	8 months pre-chemotherapy	Cycle 1	Post-cycle 3, day 28	Post-cycle 3, day 42	Cycle 5 day 16
HBV DNA	Positive: <20 IU/ml		Positive: 1.6×10^4 IU/ml	Positive: 3.6×10^4 IU/ml	Positive: <20 IU/ml
ALT	13 IU/l	20 IU/l	305 IU/l	49 IU/l	23 IU/l

Table 16.1 Results of HBV DNA and ALT tests for patient in Case History

ALT, alanine transaminase; HBV, hepatitis B virus

Describe the principles of management of hepatitis and liver failure

Reactivation of HBV can lead to acute hepatitis, fulminant liver failure and death. It is important to refer the patient to a hepatologist urgently if this is suspected or confirmed. Acute liver failure (ALF) is the rapid development of a severe acute liver injury with jaundice, coagulopathy and encephalopathy.

Patients with ALF should ideally be managed in a centre of expertise. Treatment is largely supportive, with an emphasis on the prevention of complications such as gastrointestinal bleeding from stress ulcers. The use of antivirals and the withdrawal of immunosuppressive therapy in HBV reactivation should be considered.

In some cases patients have had underlying liver disease secondary to chronic unrecognized hepatitis B, and their presentation will be one of acute or chronic liver failure, with all the incumbent complications of decompensated cirrhosis, including ascites, encephalopathy, sepsis and variceal haemorrhage.

Could this patient's chemotherapy have caused the elevated ALT and is it safe to be continued?

Changes in transaminase levels are rare with epirubicin and cyclophosphamide (EC) chemotherapy. Nevertheless, these cytotoxins should be used with extreme caution in liver disease. Epirubicin is primarily eliminated by the hepatobiliary system and therefore patients with elevated bilirubin or transaminase levels may have increased toxicity due to reduction in the drug clearance. Table 16.2 gives examples of commonly used chemotherapy drugs that are potentially hepatotoxic. Table 16.3 summarizes the chemotherapy drugs which require caution in liver disease.

Table 16.2 Examples of potentially hepatotoxic chemotherapy drugs. This information can be found in the relevant Summary of Product Characteristics (SPC)

Drug	Hepatic toxicity
Actinomycin D	Liver sinusoidal obstruction syndrome (hepatic veno-oclusive disease) is rare but potentially fatal.
Carboplatin	Abnormal liver function tests, usually transient and mild to moderate.
Gemcitabine	Mainly transient transaminitis unusual after cycle 2, reports of liver failure.
Oxaliplatin	Liver sinusoidal obstruction syndrome, common and can lead to a delay in liver resection when used in the neoadjuvant setting. Reports of acute liver failure.
Methotrexate	Significant elevations of liver enzymes, acute liver atrophy, necrosis, fatty metamorphosis, periportal fibrosis or cirrhosis or death may occur, usually following chronic administration.
Paclitaxel	Very rare, hepatic necrosis, hepatic encephalopathy (both with reported cases of fatal outcome)
Trabectedin	Abnormal liver function tests, particularly hyperbilirubinaemia. Severe hepatic injury uncommon (<1%).

Table 16.3 Chemotherapy drugs which require caution in liver disease. This information can be found in the relevant Summary of Product Characteristics (SPC).

Drug	Role of liver in metabolism	Recommendations in hepatic impairment.
Capecitabine	First metabolized in the liver but no significant role in elimination	Stop if bilirubin >3.0 × ULN or ALT, AST >2.5 × ULN occur. Resume when bilirubin decreases to ≤3.0 × ULN or ALT, AST decrease to ≤2.5 × ULN. Drug-induced haemolysis can lead to a solitary rise in bilirubin that does not require dose alteration/delay
Carboplatin	Not significant	Caution in severe liver failure
Cisplatin	Some biliary excretion	Caution in severe liver failure
Oxaliplatin	Not significant	50% dose if bilirubin >3 × ULN
Docetaxel	Mainly metabolized in the liver by cytochrome P450	Reduce dose if ALT and/or AST >1.5 × ULN concurrent with ALP >2.5 × ULN. Avoid use if bilirubin >ULN and/or ALT and AST >3.5 × ULN concurrent with serum ALP >6 times the ULN
Doxorubicin	Significant liver metabolism by cytochrome P450	50% dose if bilirubin 20–51µmol/l; 25% dose if bilirubin >51µmol/l; 75% of dose if AST 2–3 × ULN
Epirubicin	Mainly metabolized in the liver Biliary excretion: 40%	50% dose if bilirubin 20–51µmol/; 25% dose if bilirubin >51 µmol/l
Etoposide	Liver metabolized, yielding inactive metabolites	Contraindicated in severe liver failure
Fluorouracil	Partly metabolized in the liver	50% dose if bilirubin >3 × ULN or if ALT/AST >2.5 × ULN
Gemcitabine	Gemcitabine is rapidly metabolized by cytidine deaminase in the liver, kidney, blood and other tissues	80% dose if bilirubin ≥1.5 × ULN. Limited data on >5 × ULN but consider 50% dose reduction and monitor closely.
Irinotecan and active metabolites	Hepatic metabolism Biliary excretion	50% dose reduction if bilirubin 1.5-3.0 ×ULN or ALP 5 × ULN. Contraindicated if bilirubin >3 × ULN
Paclitaxel	Mainly hepatic metabolism Biliary excretion	Avoid in severe hepatic impairment (bilirubin >5 × ULN or AST/ALT >10 × ULN). Consider a dose reduction if bilirubin >2 ULN
Sorafenib	Mainly hepatic metabolism	In patients with hepatocellular carcinoma sorafenib should not be used in patients with Child Pugh score >7. Other patients: 50% dose if bilirubin >1.5-3 × ULN. Contra indicated >3 × ULN
Sunitinib	Mainly hepatic metabolism	Contra indicated if bilirubin >2 × ULN
Trabectedin	Mainly metabolized by cytochrome P450 3A4	Avoid if bilirubin elevated. Consider dose reduction if AST, ALT and/or alkaline phosphatase elevated between cycles
Vincristine	Metabolized by cytochrome P450 CYP 3A subfamily	50% dose reduction recommended if bilirubin >51 µmol/l

ALP, alkaline phosphatase; ALT, alanine transaminase; AST, aspartate transaminase; ULN, upper limit of normal

Conclusion

Disease or drug-related issues are the most common aetiology in cancer patients presenting with jaundice and can normally be managed by the multidisciplinary team. Less frequent aetiologies should still be considered and a full hepatic screen is performed in patients with hepatitic liver failure.

Patients who are currently infected with hepatitis B (HBsAg-positive) and some who have been previously infected (HBcAb-positive) are at risk of hepatitis B reactivation during immunosuppressive therapies. Hepatitis B reactivation may lead to death or significant morbidity from fulminant hepatitis and needs to be managed under specialist supervision. Treatment of reactivation necessitates interruption or cessation of chemotherapy, potentially compromising disease control. Hepatitis B reactivation can be prevented by appropriate assessment of patients for antiviral prophylaxis treatment.

Fortunately, in the case presented here a good outcome was achieved as the liver recovered quickly and radical surgery followed by adjuvant chemotherapy was still possible.

Further reading

1   Ghany M, Hoofnagle JH. Approach to the patient with liver disease. In: Longo D, Fauci A, Kasper D, Hauser S, Jameson J, Loscalzo J, editors. *Harrison's Principles of Internal Medicine.* 18th ed. McGraw-Hill; 2011. p. 2520–7.

2   Hollinger FB, Liang TJ. Hepatitis B Virus. In: Knipe DM, Howley PM, Griffin DE, *et al.*, editors. *Fields Virology.* 4th ed. Philadelphia: Lippincott Williams & Wilkins; 2001. p.2971–3036.

3   Wursthorn K, Wedemeyer H, Manns MP. Managing HBV in patients with impaired immunity. *Gut* 2010; **59**: 1430–45.

4   Katz LH, Fraser A, Gafter-Gvili A, *et al.* Lamivudine prevents reactivation of hepatitis B and reduces mortality in immunosuppressed patients: systematic review and meta-analysis. *J Viral Hepat* 2008; **15**: 89–102.

5   Yorkshire and the Humber Liver Network [Internet]. c.2013. Available from: www.yhln.org.uk

See also:

World Health Organization. [Internet]. *Hepatitis B: Introduction.* Global Alert and Response (GAR) document. World Health Organization Department of Communicable Diseases Surveillance and Response; c.2013. Available from: www.who.int/csr/disease/hepatitis/whocdscsrlyo20022/en/index1.html

PROBLEM

17 Acute Kidney Injury

Lucy Wyld, Christy Ralph, Andrew Lewington

Case History

A 76-year-old man with castrate refractory metastatic prostate cancer receiving palliative chemotherapy with docetaxel (75 mg/m² day 1, three-weekly) is admitted unwell with a two-day history of vomiting and diarrhoea following his second cycle of chemotherapy. He has a history of hypertension and hypercholesterolaemia and is taking ramipril 2.5 mg once-daily and simvastatin 20 mg at night. He weighed 68 kg and his vital signs are: temperature 37.2°C, pulse 105 bpm; blood pressure 92/60 mmHg. Urea and electrolytes: Na⁺ 136 mmol/l; K⁺ 6.5 mmol/l; urea 22 mmol/l; creatinine 245 µmol/l. Serum creatinine was 89 µmol/l two weeks previously.

What is the definition of acute kidney injury (AKI)?

What are the causes of AKI?

What are the risk factors for AKI and how can it be prevented?

What investigations should be performed in AKI?

What is the management of AKI?

What is the prognosis for AKI?

Background

What is the definition of acute kidney injury?

Acute kidney injury (AKI) can be considered a spectrum of injury, with even relatively minor rises in serum creatinine being associated with an increased morbidity and mortality. Recent definitions have been based upon rises in serum creatinine or falls in urine output and have been harmonized by the international guideline organization, Kidney Diseases: Improving Global Outcomes (KDIGO).

Acute kidney injury is defined when one of the following criteria is met:

- Serum creatinine rises by 26 µmol/l within 48 hours;
- Serum creatinine rises 1.5-fold from the reference value,* which is known or presumed to have occurred within 1 week;
- Urine output is <0.5 ml/kg for more than six consecutive hours.

*The reference serum creatinine should be the lowest creatinine value recorded within 3 months of the event.

Patients with cancer may have a reduced muscle mass (sarcopenia) which can be a consequence of both cancer cachexia and treatment (e.g. with tyrosine kinase inhibitors). The result is a low baseline level of serum creatinine and the potential to overestimate the patient's kidney function, which may then lead to incorrect drug dosing. Such patients will have a reduced functional kidney reserve and be at risk of AKI.

Table 17.1 Causes of acute kidney injury (AKI)

Classification of AKI	Cause
Prerenal (functional process)	Acute heart failure
	Liver failure (hepatorenal failure)
	Sepsis
	Hypovolaemia (diarrhoea, mucositis, vomiting, interleukin-2, hypercalcaemia)
	Nephrotoxins (aminoglycosides, non-steroidal anti-inflammatory drugs, iodinated contrast)
Renal (damage to renal vasculature, nephron or interstitium)	**Vascular:** haemolytic uraemic syndrome/thrombotic thrombocytopenic pupura (adenocarcinoma of stomach, pancreas or prostate, mitomycin, gemcitabine, bleomycin and cisplatin combination therapy, VEGF inhibitors) renal artery/vein thrombosis,
	Glomerulonephritis: membranous nephropathy (solid tumours), minimal change nephropathy (Hodgkin's lymphoma), crescentic glomerulonephritis (ANCA-associated vasculitis), focal segmental glomerulosclerosis (iv bisphosphonates)
	Acute tubular injury: rhabdomyolysis, tumour lysis syndrome, iodinated contrast and drugs (e.g. methotrexate, cisplatin, bisphosphonates, tyrosine kinase inhibitors, ifosfamide, aminoglycosides)
	Interstitial nephritis: drugs (NSAIDs, β-lactam antibiotics, diuretics), infection and systemic disease (sarcoid, lymphoma, leukaemia)
	Amyloidosis: myeloma, renal cell carcinoma, Hodgkin's lymphoma, chronic lymphocytic leukaemia
	Light chain deposition disease: myeloma, Waldenstrom macroglobulinaemia
	Myeloma cast nephropathy
	Tumour infiltration: lymphoma, acute leukaemia
Post-renal	**Ureteric obstruction:** stone disease, tumour, fibrosis, ligation post pelvic surgery
	Bladder neck obstruction: benign prostatic hypertrophy, prostate cancer, neurogenic bladder, bladder tumour, blood clots, retroperitoneal fibrosis, colon cancer and lymphoma
	Urethral obstruction: strictures, tumour
	Intra-abdominal hypertension: tense ascites

ANCA, antineutrophil cytoplasmic antibody; NSAID, non-steroidal anti-inflammatory drug; VEGF, vascular endothelial growth factor

The recognition of AKI may be hampered because the reduced muscle mass and creatinine production will limit the rise in serum creatinine and mask the severity of the underlying injury.

What are the causes of AKI?

When a diagnosis of AKI is made it is essential to ascertain the cause as that will allow appropriate, prompt treatment (Table 17.1). The most common causes include sepsis, hypovolaemia and nephrotoxins, but AKI may also develop secondary to complications from oncological treatments or the disease process itself.

What are the risk factors for AKI and how can it be prevented?

The prevention of AKI is an important part of care for all patients with cancer. It is essential that risk factors for AKI (Table 17.2) are identified early and appropriate measures taken, such as prompt treatment of sepsis, rapid correction of hypovolaemia and avoidance of nephrotoxins.

Table 17.2 AKI risk factors
Age >75 yrs
Chronic kidney disease (eGFR <60 ml/min/1.73m^2)
Atherosclerotic peripheral vascular disease
Liver disease
Diabetes mellitus
Cardiac failure
Nephrotoxins (e.g. NSAIDS, cisplatin, iodinated contrast)
Sepsis
Hypovolaemia

Tumour lysis syndrome (TLS) results from severe hyperuricaemia and tubular obstruction with uric acid crystals and/or calcium phosphate. It can occur following initiation of therapy for high-grade lymphomas or acute lymphoblastic leukaemia, but may also be a spontaneous phenomenon in some tumours. The risk of AKI can be reduced by intravenous volume expansion and administration of rasburicase (xanthine oxidase inhibitor).

Computed tomography (CT) with iodinated contrast has become a routine part of chemotherapy response assessment in many cancers. The risk of contrast-induced acute kidney injury (CI-AKI) is significantly higher in patients with underlying chronic kidney disease (CKD). It is therefore important to identify patients at risk and consider whether the clinical information obtained from CT will outweigh the risk of CI-AKI. Strategies to reduce the incidence of CI-AKI include intravenous volume expansion pre- and post-CT, avoidance of nephrotoxic medications and minimizing the dose of iodinated contrast.

What investigations should be performed in AKI?

Appropriate baseline investigations include serum urea and electrolytes ('U&Es') and full blood count, with the addition of urine and blood cultures if sepsis is suspected. A urinalysis should be performed and a renal tract ultrasound within 24 hours is warranted if obstruction is suspected.

What is the management of AKI?

Any patient presenting with AKI should have a comprehensive history and examination performed, which should include the identification of AKI risk factors (Table 17.2) and potential causes (Table 17.1). The patient's volume status must be carefully assessed, involving the following: capillary refill, pulse rate, blood pressure, jugular venous pressure, skin turgor, presence of oedema (pulmonary and peripheral), and also evaluating fluid balance charts, urine output and daily weights.

Patients receiving intravenous fluids should be monitored closely with regular volume status evaluation, daily U&Es, and have appropriate end-points determined. Nutritional support should be considered in all patients with AKI, with a recommended intake of 25–30 kcal/kg/day. Sepsis must be considered and treated for promptly in all patients with AKI.

The indication and dose of all medications in patients with AKI should be reviewed. Nephrotoxic medications such as NSAIDs and aminoglycosides should be withheld or avoided. Patients with AKI secondary to medication will require cessation of the offending drug.

Bladder outflow obstruction can be relieved with the placement of a bladder catheter. However, there needs to be careful consideration of bleeding risk (due to potential abnormalities in clotting factors and/or platelets) and antibiotic cover may be necessary if neutropenia is possible (avoid gentamicin). Upper urinary tract obstruction secondary to cancer will require urology or interventional radiology input and consideration of a ureteric stent insertion or percutaneous nephrostomy. This decision will be based on the patient's wishes, the nature of the obstruction, the chance of resolution with chemotherapy and the risk of urinary sepsis.

Referral to nephrology is recommended early if the cause of AKI is not easily explained and rarer forms are suspected. Referral is also recommended if the AKI is progressive in the setting of oliguria, or if complications occur that are refractory to medical therapy. Complications might include metabolic acidosis, hyperkalaemia, pulmonary oedema, or uraemic symptoms such as encephalopathy and pericarditis.

What is the prognosis of AKI?

There is a lack of cancer-specific data detailing the prognosis in patients with AKI. Mortality rates can vary between 10% and 80%. However, it is becoming clearer that in patients with AKI it is the severity and duration of the episode that predicts progressive CKD. The development of CKD in patients with cancer has important implications for the dosing and safety of future chemotherapy, analgesia, antibiotics and imaging techniques (especially iodinated contrast) used, and may subsequently affect the success of further active anticancer treatment.

Conclusion

 Acute kidney injury is a syndrome which has many different causes and is often multifactorial in patients with cancer. It is important to identify risk factors for AKI and institute preventative measures wherever possible. Effective management is dependent upon early recognition and correction of hypovolaemia, as well as promptly addressing reversible causes, such as sepsis and withdrawal of nephrotoxins. It is now recognized that the severity and duration of AKI predicts the progression to CKD, which has important implications for patients with cancer.

Further reading

1 Drumi W. Nutritional management of acute renal failure. *J Renal Nutrition* 2005; **15**: 63–70.

2 Espinel CH, Gregory AW. Differential diagnosis of acute renal failure. *Clin Nephrol* 1980; **13**: 73–7.

3 Kidney Disease: Improving Global Outcomes (KDIGO) Acute Kidney Injury Work Group. KDIGO Clinical Practice Guideline for Acute Kidney Injury. *Kidney Inter Suppl* 2012; **2**: 1–138.

4 Lamiere NH, Flombaum CD, Moreau D, Ronco C. Acute renal failure in cancer patients. *Ann Med* 2005; **37**: 13–25.

5 Lewington A, Kanagasundaram S. Renal Association Clinical Practice Guidelines on acute kidney injury. *Nephron Clin Pract* 2011; **118**: 349–90.

6 Lines S, Lewington A. Acute kidney injury. *Clin Med* 2009; **9**(3): 273–7.

7 Praught ML, Shiplak MG. Are small changes in serum creatinine an important risk factor? *Curr Opin Nephrol Hypertens* 2005; **14**: 265–70.

8 Sahni V, Choudhury D, Ahmed Z, *et al.* Chemotherapy-associated renal dysfunction. *Nat Rev Nephrol* 2009; **5**: 450–62.

18 Chemotherapy-Related Renal Toxicity

Lucy Wyld, Christy Ralph, Andrew Lewington

Case History

A 57-year-old man presents with metastatic transitional cell cancer of the upper urinary tract causing solitary hydronephrosis and flank pain. He has a history of severe anxiety and is taking amitriptyline 200 mg once daily and ibuprofen 400 mg thrice daily. The patient's weight is 62 kg. His urea and electrolytes are: Na⁺ 138 mmol/l; K⁺ 5.3 mmol/l; urea 4.0 mmol/l; creatinine 108 μmol/l; eGFR 61 ml/min/1.73m². His Eastern Cooperative Oncology Group (ECOG) performance status (PS) is 1 and he is keen to proceed with palliative chemotherapy.

What are the risk factors for chemotherapy-related renal toxicity?

Can we estimate renal function accurately?

Which chemotherapy drugs are commonly associated with renal toxicity?

What steps can be taken to prevent chemotherapy-related renal toxicity?

What are the long-term consequences?

Background

What are the risk factors for chemotherapy-related renal toxicity?

Toxicity from chemotherapy can cause both acute kidney injury (AKI) and chronic kidney disease (CKD). The diagnosis and management of AKI is discussed in Chapter 17. This chapter will focus on the recognition of the 'at-risk' patient and the adaptations required in their oncology management.

Key risk factors for chemotherapy-related renal toxicity are:

- Age >75 yrs
- Pre-existing chronic kidney disease (CKD) eGFR <60 ml/min/1.73m²
- Hypoalbuminaemia (alters drug handling)
- Choice of chemotherapy
- Hypovolaemia, e.g. vomiting, diuretics
- Concomitant use of other nephrotoxins, e.g. NSAIDs, aminoglycosides, iodinated contrast
- Urinary tract obstruction.

Can we estimate renal function accurately?

Many chemotherapy drugs are excreted by the kidneys via either glomerular filtration or tubular secretion. Where the drug and/or its active metabolites are excreted by the kidneys, an estimation of renal function is essential to ensure safe dosing of treatment. Unfortunately, serum creatinine is a poor biomarker of renal function in patients with cancer due to a reduced muscle mass (sarcopenia). Equations such as the Cockcroft–Gault formula, modification of diet in renal disease (MDRD) formula or Wright formula use serum creatinine to calculate renal function and therefore have the potential to overestimate the glomerular filtration rate (GFR) in patients with cancer. The gold standard investigation for renal function remains an isotope GFR and should be used to ensure safe treatment of those patients where estimated GFR is in doubt.

Which chemotherapy drugs are commonly associated with renal toxicity?

Many drugs used to treat malignant disease have the potential to cause renal toxicity and electrolyte disturbances. The drugs can exert their toxic effects either directly or indirectly, the latter as a consequence of sepsis or other severe toxicity such as mucositis or diarrhoea. The details of chemotherapy-related renal toxicity and mechanisms are outside the scope of this review but should be considered by the treating physician. However a brief review of common exemplar drugs can be found in Table 18.1.

What steps can be taken to prevent chemotherapy–related renal toxicity?

Nephrotoxicity is an inherent adverse effect of certain anticancer drugs. The most important step in reducing the risk of nephrotoxicity lies in thorough clinical assessment and monitoring. Avoidance, early detection and treatment can prevent the development of cumulative kidney damage which may, in turn, result in progressive CKD.

Assessment
- Identify at-risk patients.
- Give appropriate consideration to the risk/benefit of treatment and potential alternatives.
- Modify choice of chemotherapy drug.
- Adjust chemotherapy dosage according to the patient's renal function.
- Review supportive and regular medications; avoid co-administration of nephrotoxic drugs.
- Assess and optimize volume status prior to starting chemotherapy.
- Measure baseline bloods, including, urea, creatinine, electrolytes and magnesium.
- Estimate (+/- measure) GFR.

Safety and monitoring
- Ensure continuous close monitoring of patient's volume status and appropriate administration of intravenous fluids.
- Monitor urea, creatinine and electrolytes with an estimate of GFR at least every cycle, but also consider additional mid-cycle safety blood tests.
- Repeat weighing with each cycle and recalculate GFR and drug dose.
- Closely monitor potassium and magnesium levels and supplement when necessary.
- Administer effective antiemetic drugs to avoid dehydration.

- Ensure early recognition and treatment of chemotherapy-induced diarrhoea.
- Educate patient about the risks of dehydration, and provide advice regarding appropriate telephone advice and triage review.

What are the long-term consequences?

There is a paucity of data surrounding the outcomes of patients who experience renal toxicity. It is important to remember that serum creatinine is a poor biomarker of renal damage. Gradual rises in serum creatinine may signify subclinical damage, for which there are many causes. Newer biomarkers are required to allow more careful monitoring of renal function and appropriate modification of therapy.

Conclusion

Many anticancer therapies are associated with renal toxicity. The mechanisms underlying kidney damage are diverse and the resultant clinical syndromes insidious. It is important to assess all patients for risk factors for AKI and tailor the treatment to the patient. Accurate and frequent evaluation of the patient, their blood tests and their volume status may allow early detection and treatment of CKD and thus prevent the long-term sequelae of chemotherapy-induced nephrotoxicity.

Further reading

1   Drumi W. Nutritional management of acute renal failure. *J Renal Nutrition* 2005; **15**: 63–70.

2   Espinel CH, Gregory AW. Differential diagnosis of acute renal failure. *Clin Nephrol* 1980; **13**: 73–7.

3   Kidney Disease: Improving Global Outcomes (KDIGO) Acute Kidney Injury Work Group. KDIGO Clinical Practice Guideline for Acute Kidney Injury. *Kidney Int Suppl* 2012; **2**: 1–138.

4   Lamiere NH, Flombaum CD, Moreau D, Ronco C. Acute renal failure in cancer patients. *Ann Med* 2005; **37**: 13–25.

5   Lewington A, Kanagasundaram S. Renal Association Clinical Practice Guidelines on acute kidney injury. *Nephron Clin Pract* 2011; **118**: 349–90.

6   Lines S, Lewington A. Acute kidney injury. *Clin Med* 2009; **9**(3): 273–7.

7   Praught ML, Shiplak MG. Are small changes in serum creatinine an important risk factor? *Curr Opin Nephrol Hypertens* 2005; **14**: 265–70.

8   Sahni V, Choudhury D, Ahmed Z, *et al.* Chemotherapy-associated renal dysfunction. *Nat Rev Nephrol* 2009; **5**: 450–62.

Table 18.1 Drugs commonly associated with renal toxicity

Drug	Renal toxicity	Management considerations
Cisplatin	Nephrotoxicity occurs in one-third of patients Associated with AKI and CKD Results in inability to concentrate urine and magnesium wasting.	Adequate pre and post hydration Magnesium monitoring and replacement Consider stopping or dose reduction
Carboplatin	Significantly less nephrotoxic than cisplatin	Dose based on renal function and area under the curve (AUC) Close monitoring of patient weight and renal function required
Cyclophosphamide	Haemorrhagic cystitis (direct toxic effect) Hyponatraemia (increased ADH activity)	Mesna is effective in the prevention of haemorrhagic cystitis Renal impairment is usually self-limiting
Capecitabine	Moderate renal impairment leads to an increase in severe capecitabine toxicities. Unlike 5-fluorouracil, capecitabine is largely excreted by the kidneys.	Dose reduction required in renal impairment Administration is contraindicated in patients with creatinine clearance <30 ml/min
Ifosfamide	Occurs in up to 30% of patients. Decreased GFR Haemorrhagic cystitis Hyponatraemia	Mesna is effective in preventing haemorrhagic cystitis but not the renal tubular injury In event of nephrotoxicity, consider dose reduction or cessation of ifosfamide Replace electrolytes
Bevacizumab (monoclonal anti-VEGF antibody)	Hypertension Proteinuria Rarely progresses to nephrotic syndrome >3.5 g proteinuria/24 h with or without clinical nephrotic syndrome (2%)	Close monitoring of kidney function, blood pressure and urinary protein excretion
VEGF inhibitors (e.g. sunitinib, sorafenib)	Hypertension	Prompt treatment of hypertension

ADH, antidiuretic hormone; AKI, acute kidney injury; CKD, chronic kidney disease

19 Metabolic Complications

Emma Rathbone, Jennifer Walsh, Janet Brown

Case History

A 52-year-old woman with metastatic renal cell carcinoma including lung metastases, and currently on sunitinib therapy, was admitted to the acute oncology unit with a one-week history of increasing shortness of breath and bilateral ankle swelling. On questioning, she described a three-week history of fatigue that was limiting her daily activities, and she was additionally now troubled with constipation. The differential diagnosis included progressive renal cell carcinoma, cardiac failure (possible secondary to her sunitinib therapy) or pulmonary embolus.

On examination the patient had dry skin, bilateral leg oedema to the mid calf, and periorbital oedema. She was bradycardic and had a respiratory rate of 24 breaths per minute. Her chest was dull to percussion to the level of the mid-zones with decreased breath sounds bilaterally.

An electrocardiogram (ECG) confirmed bradycardia, rate 45 beats per minute (bpm); a chest X-ray confirmed bilateral pleural effusions and the known pulmonary metastases, which appeared unchanged compared to previous films. Full blood count was normal, with mild hyponatraemia (130 mmol/l) on urea and electrolyte tests ('U&Es'), and normal liver function. She was initially managed with oxygen therapy and drainage of pleural fluid. Subsequent thyroid function tests revealed overt hypothyroidism with thyroid-stimulating hormone (TSH) 42 milliunits per litre (mIU/l; reference range 0.2–6.0 mIU/l) and free thyroxine (T4) of 5.6 pmol/l (reference range 10–25 pmol/l). She was commenced on thyroxine 25 µg/day.

What is the cause of this patient's thyroid dysfunction?

How would you manage this patient?

What other conditions may present with similar features?

What are the new developments with regards to treatment with tyrosine kinase inhibitors?

What other metabolic complications may be caused by systemic anticancer therapy?

Background

What is the cause of this patient's thyroid dysfunction?

A number of cancer therapies are known to lead to thyroid dysfunction. These include interferon and interleukin, as well as newer targeted therapies such as tyrosine kinase inhibitors (TKIs), which include sunitinib, pazopanib and sorafenib, that are used in a range of cancers. For example, sunitinib is a TKI licensed for use in renal cell carcinoma, gastrointestinal stromal tumours (GIST) and pancreatic neuroendocrine tumours. As a class, TKIs are known to cause thyroid dysfunction through different mechanisms. It has been proposed that sunitinib may prevent vascular endothelial growth factor (VEGF) from binding to normal thyroid cells (resulting in loss of capillary circulation), reduce synthesis of thyroid hormones (through decreased iodine uptake or decreased peroxidise activity), or cause destructive thyroiditis.[1] These agents are likely to worsen pre-existing hypothyroidism as well as cause a newly developed condition. Sunitinib can induce hypothyroidism in 36%–85% of patients, whilst sorafenib and pazopanib present a slightly lower incidence.[1–3] Most thyroid dysfunction associated with TKI use is asymptomatic biochemical subclinical hypothyroidism (this means raised TSH, with thyroid hormones within the reference range), and abnormalities of thyroid function tests may be transient. Thyroid auto-antibodies are usually negative.

It has been reported that the duration of treatment with TKI is an important risk factor for the development of hypothyroidism. For example, Desai *et al.* (2006) reported that in patients on sunitinib for GIST 18% developed hypothyroidism by 36 weeks, 29% by 52 weeks, and 90% if duration of use was greater than 96 weeks.[4] The mean time to development of hypothyroidism was 50 weeks.

Although the condition is often subclinical, symptoms may occur either insidiously or, less commonly, with overt hypothyroidism. Common presenting features may be fatigue, slow cognition, weight gain, cold intolerance, constipation, shortness of breath, peripheral oedema, and skin and hair changes.

How would you manage this patient?

Any acute manifestations (e.g. pericardial or pleural effusions) should be treated as a matter of priority according to usual medical management. Thyroid replacement therapy (levothyroxine) is the mainstay of treatment (usually titrated up from 25–50 µg daily) and should ideally involve shared care with the GP. Treatment with thyroxine should be considered in patients with thyroid hormones below the lower limit of the reference range, or with normal thyroid hormones but TSH levels >10 mIU/l, or symptoms likely to be due to hypothyroidism.

In most cases, treatment with the TKI can continue with careful management of thyroid function.

What other conditions may present with similar features?

Fatigue related to cancer or treatment for cancer may present similarly, and indeed may be difficult to distinguish from symptoms due to hypothyroidism. Additionally, progressive malignant disease should be considered, as there are several overlapping complaints (e.g. increasing fatigue, fluid retention, decreasing performance status) and the two conditions may coexist. Treatment with TKIs can also be directly cardiotoxic, causing left ventricular dysfunction, congestive heart failure and arrhythmias. Finally, depression should be considered, as this is common in cancer patients, though frequently under-reported.

Recent Developments

What are the new developments with regard to treatment with tyrosine kinase inhibitors?

As newer TKIs are developed, and the scope of use for those already established widens, it is of great importance that algorithms are produced to guide monitoring and replacement therapy. A proposed guideline has already been published and will be a useful aid to clinicians caring for patients on these drugs.[1] The guideline recommends baseline thyroid function tests and different management for subclinical versus overt hypothyroidism, with repeat TSH measurement on day one of every cycle.

It is now reported that the newer second-generation TKIs, including dasatinib and nilotinib, also cause thyroid dysfunction.[5] It is likely that patients may experience more than one line of therapy with TKIs, possibly moving from one to another through the course of their management, with the potential risk of cumulative toxicity. Whether there is any additive effect on the thyroid remains unknown, but will certainly require continued close monitoring of thyroid function.

Conclusion

Clinicians need to be aware of the potential for thyroid dysfunction with newer targeted therapies. Often symptoms can be very similar to disease progression and, of course, both may be present. Monitoring of thyroid function allows identification and treatment of patients who are developing overt hypothyroidism.

What other metabolic complications may be caused by systemic anticancer therapy?

There are many other metabolic complications of anticancer drugs to consider in an acutely presenting cancer patient. Table 19.1 summarizes the most common ones.

Further reading

1   Torino F, Corsello SM, Longo R, Barnabei A, Gasparini G. Hypothyroidism related to tyrosine kinase inhibitors: an emerging toxic effect of targeted therapy. *Nat Rev Clin Oncol* 2009; **6**(4): 219–28.

2   Clemons J, Gao D, Naam M, Breaker K, Garfield D, Flaig TW. Thyroid dysfunction in patients treated with sunitinib or sorafenib. *Clin Genitourin Cancer* 2012; **10**(4): 225–31.

3   Eisen T, Sternberg CN, Robert C, *et al.* Targeted therapies for renal cell carcinoma: review of adverse event management strategies. *J Natl Cancer Inst* 2012; **104**(2): 93–113.

4   Desai J, Yassa L, Marqusee E, *et al.* Hypothyroidism after sunitinib treatment for patients with gastrointestinal stromal tumors. *Ann Intern Med* 2006; **145**(9): 660–4.

5   Kim TD, Schwarz M, Nogai H, *et al.* Thyroid dysfunction caused by second-generation tyrosine kinase inhibitors in Philadelphia chromosome-positive chronic myeloid leukemia. *Thyroid* 2010; **20**(11): 1209–14.

See also:

Brown RL. Tyrosine kinase inhibitor-induced hypothyroidism: incidence, etiology, and management. *Target Oncol* 2011; **6**(4): 217–26.

Table 19.1 Metabolic complications caused by systemic chemotherapy

Complication	Example responsible drug	Presenting symptoms	Treatment considerations
Hyponatraemia	Cisplatin (salt-wasting) Cylophosphamide (SIADH)	Anorexia, nausea, asthenia, seizures, hypotonia, coma	Assess fluid balance status and measure serum and urine sodium and osmolality to ensure accurate diagnosis of cause of hyponatraemia and guide treatment.
Hypomagnesaemia	Cisplatin Aminoglycosides	Increased neuromuscular excitability, seizures, cardiac arrhythmias, likely to be accompanied by low Ca	Replace Mg. Rapidly developing , severe or significantly symptomatic hypomagnesaemia requires more rapid replacement than milder hypomagnesaemia.
Hypocalcaemia	Cisplatin, bisphosphonates, denosumab	Tingling fingers, tremors, tetany, seizures, cardiac arrhythmias	As for hypomagnesaemia. In an emergency 10 ml 10% calcium gluconate IV over 30 min. Repeat as necessary.
Hyperuricaemia	Cisplatin, etoposide. May be part of tumour lysis syndrome	Acute kidney injury	Rehydration. Consider haemodialysis in severe cases. Allopurinol to prevent.
Adrenal suppression	Withdrawal of steroids e.g. dexamethasone	Fatigue, hypoglycaemia, hyponatraemia, nausea, vomiting, hypotension (adrenal crisis)	Rehydration, IV hydrocortisone 100 mg qds. Can be prevented by slowly reducing dose.

IV, intravenous; qds, four times a day; SIADH, syndrome of inappropriate antidiuretic hormone secretion

20 Diabetes

Jenny Seligmann, Dan Swinson, Stephen Gilbey

Case History

A female patient with poorly controlled type 2 (non-insulin dependent) diabetes mellitus (DM) presented with pulmonary metastases from a colon cancer, three years after right hemicolectomy and adjuvant chemotherapy.

The patient was initially managed expectantly; on progression she remained fit, performance status 0, isotope GFR 72 ml/min, and was treated with irinotecan/5-fluorouracil/bevacizumab within a clinical trial for first line treatment.

Immediate complications occurred, with two Hickman line infections requiring intravenous antibiotics and line replacement, and a further admission with acute kidney injury (AKI) attributed to NSAIDs, all prior to cycle 3. Control insulin was initiated and chemotherapy paused to try and improve DM control. One month later the patient was admitted from clinic with septis due to a retroperitoneal abscess. After drainage and protracted antibiotics, her recovery was complicated by *Clostridium difficile* diarrhoea.

Five months after the two cycles of chemotherapy, the patient was reviewed in clinic: she had chosen to revert to oral hypoglycaemic drugs, and a CT scan showed disease control of the colon cancer.

The patient's disease progressed two months later and she was re-challenged with reduced dose irinotecan and capecitabine every two weeks (to avoid an indwelling line). Following the second cycle she was admitted with necrotising fasciitis of the scalp, which required surgical debridement and protracted antibiotics. Chemotherapy was stopped. The patient died four months later from acute bowel ischaemia.

What risks does a diagnosis of diabetes mellitus pose to a cancer patient?

Can cancer patients with diabetes mellitus be risk stratified?

Should patients with diabetes mellitus be managed differently?

Background

The prevalence of DM (366 million worldwide in 2011) increases with age and reaches 15% in the 60–79-year-old age bracket. A significant proportion of patients remain undiagnosed.[1] In general, these diabetic patients have a 20% higher risk of hospital admission and 10% higher in-hospital mortality, after adjusting for confounding factors.[1] Patients with diabetes are at increased risk of infection and there is a doubling of infection-related mortality.[2,3] Diabetic patients are also at higher risk of some types of solid organ cancers.[4]

What risks does a diagnosis of diabetes mellitus pose to a cancer patient?

During the management of potentially curative treatment DM has been found to be associated with:

- increased post-operative mortality in colorectal cancer patients
- lower likelihood of being offered adjuvant chemotherapy
- increased risk of diarrhoea following adjuvant fluoropyrimidine chemotherapy
- increased risk of hospital admission following adjuvant chemotherapy for breast cancer due to toxicity and infection.

Less information is available on the impact of DM on the management of advanced cancers. At the St James's Institute of Oncology (SJIO), a retrospective cohort study was conducted comparing diabetic patients treated for advanced colorectal cancer and gynaecological cancers from 2001 to 11 during their first 18 weeks of chemotherapy.[5] Diabetes was associated with:

- A three fold increase in acute admissions (41% infective, 17% poor glycaemic control)
- A two fold increase in the early stopping of chemotherapy
- A reduced use of second line chemotherapy.

Can cancer patients with diabetes mellitus be risk stratified?

This area has not been investigated in any detail in non-surgical cancer patients.

A long-term marker of glycaemic control is HbA1c level, and a value over 60 mmol/mol predicts an increased risk of both hyper- and hypoglycaemia. There is mixed evidence linking high HbA1c levels with risk of post-operative complications following various surgical procedures.

Evidence of end-organ damage may increase risk: a study of patients undergoing foot surgery found an increased risk of infection was limited to DM patients with a peripheral neuropathy.[6]

Should patients with diabetes mellitus be managed differently?

Chemotherapy

Oncologists should be aware of the increased risks of complications in DM patients. Limited evidence is available to guide management. At the SJIO an algorithm has been developed to guide practice based on core principles and is centred on joint working between oncology and diabetic care teams (Figure 20.1 and Table 20.1).

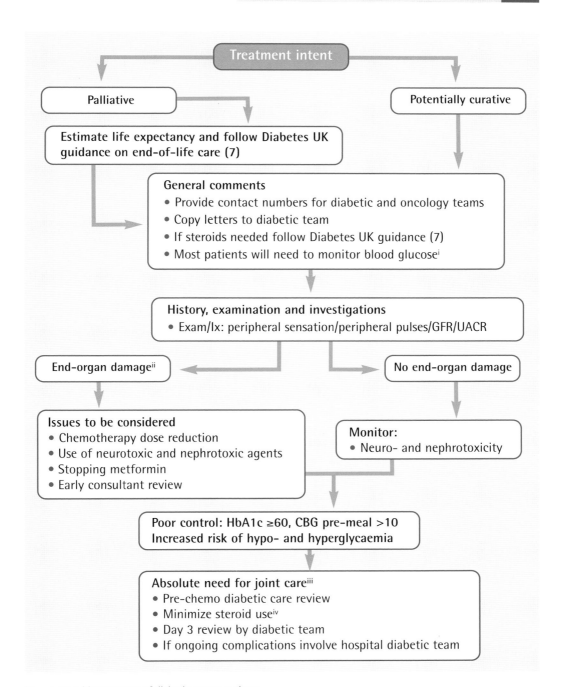

Figure 20.1 Management of diabetic cancer patients

i Blood glucose monitoring will need to be initiated if steroids are required.
ii GFR<50, peripheral neuropathy, ischaemic heart disease or retinopathy.
iii Oncology and primary or secondary care diabetic team.
iv Consider omitting day 2–5 dexamethasone if no acute emesis or substitute (see Table 20.1).

Table 20.1 Alternative antiemetics to corticosteroids	
Drug	Type of emesis
5HT3 antagonists	Immediate emesis
Neurokinin receptor antagonists	Immediate and delayed emesis
Olanzepine*	Immediate and delayed emesis
Metoclopramide or domperidone	Delayed emesis

*Perturbations of blood sugar listed as common in Summary of Product Characteristics and therefore should also be used with caution.

Modifications and cautions with hypoglycaemic agents
- Stop metformin:
  prior to and 48 hours after administration of iodinated contrast agents
  if glomerular filtration rate (GFR) <35 ml/min/1.73 m² hypoxia, sepsis, hepatic failure (clinical syndrome, raised INR attributable) or heart failure.
- Stop GLP-1 analogs (liraglutide, exenatide) if GFR <35 ml/min/1.73 m².
- Dose reduce DPP-4 inhibitors (sitagliptin, vildagliptin, saxagliptin) if GFR <35 ml/min/1.73 m².
- Consider dose reduction following fall in renal function for patients on sulfonylureas (e.g. gliclazide) or insulin due to risk of hypoglycaemia.

Management of acutely ill diabetes patients with or without acute hyperglycaemia
The principles are as for any diabetes emergency:
- Hydration
- Glucose control
- Assessment of ketonuria, acidosis, and requirement for insulin – local guidelines may vary depending on whether the patient has ketoacidosis or hyperglycaemic hyperosmolar state
- Close monitoring of cardiovascular status
- Exclusion of complicating factors such as infection, gastroparesis
- The use of pumped intravenous insulin following local hospital guidelines
- Involvement of the inpatient hospital diabetes team at an early stage if there is any suggestion of metabolic decompensation, and the clinical situation is deteriorating despite the application of clinical guidelines and protocols.

The local specialist diabetes team will be aware of the local pathways for management and will be in a position to assess whether a patient can revert to community care on discharge or needs to be followed up by the hospital diabetes service.

End-of-life care
Diabetes UK has developed guidelines for management of end-of-life care for patients with diabetes.[7] The general principles are to use the simplest and least intrusive treatment regimen to maintain comfort and quality of life, with no consideration for overall diabetes care. In many cases where active treatment is needed, it will prove easier to rely on a

simplified insulin regimen than to continue with a panoply of oral medications. This implies that the patient, their carers, or the community clinical teams can monitor glucose appropriately and coordinate adjustments to insulin treatment specifically to avoid hypoglycaemia.

Conclusion

Diabetic cancer patients are at higher risk of chemotherapy-related toxicity. Failure to include due consideration of a diagnosis of diabetes and associated pathology may result in unnecessary complications and curtailment of treatment. There are limited data to guide management. Empirically, we would recommend a low threshold for upfront dose reductions for diabetic patients with raised HbA1c (>60 mmol/mol) or end-organ damage. Joint management of these patients with the diabetic services should be a core principle.

Further reading

1   National Diabetes Information Service. *NHS Atlas of Variation in Healthcare for People with Diabetes: Reducing unwarranted variation to increase value and improve quality.* NHS Right Care; Jun 2012. 100p. Available from: www.rightcare.nhs.uk/index.php/atlas/diabetes

2   Muller LM, Gorter KJ, Hak E *et al.* Increased risk of common infections in patients with type 1 and type 2 diabetes mellitus. *Clin Infect Dis* 2005; **41**: 281–8.

3   Shah B, Hux JE. Quantifying the risk of infectious diseases for people with diabetes. *Diabetes Care* 2003; **26**: 510–13.

4   Johnson JA, Carstensen B, Witte D, *et al.* Diabetes and cancer (1): evaluating the temporal relationship between type 2 diabetes and cancer incidence. *Diabetologia* 2012; **55**:1607–18.

5   Seligmann J, Young A, Heath G, *et al.* [Abstract 1549PD] Treating diabetic patients with chemotherapy: single centre experience of toxicity and outcomes. *Ann Oncol* 2012; **23** (suppl 9): ix499–ix527.

6   Wukich DK, Lowery NJ, McMillen RL, *et al.* Postoperative infection rates in foot and ankle surgery: a comparison of patients with and without diabetes mellitus. *J Bone Joint Surg Am* 2010; **92**: 287–95.

7   Diabetes UK. *End Of Life Diabetes Care: Clinical Care Recommendations.* London: Diabetes UK; Jul 2012. 24pp. Available from: www.diabetes.org.uk/About_us/Position-statements—recommendations/Position-statements/End-of-Life-Care-/

PROBLEM

21 Cutaneous Manifestations of Chemotherapy

Mehran Afshar, Cath Siller, Julia Newton Bishop

Case History

A 54-year-old woman with metastatic breast cancer receiving capecitabine chemotherapy calls the Acute Oncology Admissions Unit, complaining of a worsening 'rash' affecting her hands and feet. She describes cracks in her skin which appear infected, and she cannot walk because of pain.

What is hand–foot syndrome and how is it described?

How is hand–foot syndrome managed?

What are the other common cutaneous side effects of chemotherapy?

Background

What is hand–foot syndrome and how is it described?

The patient had noticed the skin changes eight days after starting her second cycle of capecitabine, and had experienced some minor changes at the end of her first cycle, but did not mention it to her oncologist. The most likely cause for the rash in this case is hand–foot syndrome (HFS). Hand–foot syndrome is one of the more common skin reactions to chemotherapy and is known by several other names: acral erythema, toxic erythema of the palms and soles, and palmar, plantar erythrodysesthesia. It is most commonly seen as a complication of capecitabine and fluorouracil, although pegylated liposomal doxorubicin, cisplatin, docetaxel, paclitaxel, methotrexate, sunitinib, sorafenib and several other drugs have also been implicated.[1,2] Although the mechanism is not fully understood, studies have shown increased Ki-67 enzyme activity in the palms compared with the skin of the back, indicating increased basal cell proliferation in this area. Additionally, expression of the activating enzyme thymidine phosphorylase is significantly elevated in the skin of the palms of the hands compared to the back, suggesting potential explanations for the origin of capecitabine-related HFS.

The clinical picture is of a progressive symmetrical erythema that is most pronounced overlying the fat pads of the distal phalanges, and often preceded by an initial complaint of tingling in the palms and soles. The erythema may spread, then blister and desquamate. The skin may crack, particularly in the natural anatomical creases or the heels, and infection may be introduced. Pain in the affected areas is common and may lead to functional disturbance.

Inability to perform activities of daily living (ADLs) as a result of pain is one of the factors in the Common Terminology Criteria for Adverse Events (CTCAE) grading criteria used to describe HFS (Table 21.1).[3]

Table 21.1	NCI Common Terminology Criteria for Adverse Events (CTCAE) grading scale for hand-foot syndrome.
Grade	Symptoms and signs
1	Minimal skin changes or dermatitis (e.g. erythema, oedema or hyperkeratosis) without pain.
2	Skin changes (e.g. peeling, blisters, bleeding, oedema or hyperkeratosis) with pain which limits instrumental ADLs.
3	Severe skin changes (e.g. peeling, blisters, bleeding, oedema or hyperkeratosis) with pain, limiting self-care ADLs.

ADLs, activities of daily living; NCI, National Cancer Institute

Recent Developments

How is hand–foot syndrome managed?
The primary objectives in the management of HFS include early detection and prevention of progression to CTCAE grade 3 symptoms. Figure 21.1 illustrates the management of HFS in patients with metastatic disease receiving capecitabine treatment.[4]

Symptomatic and supportive measures, such as the use of simple emollients, adequate analgesia, and antibiotic treatment for secondary infection, should be considered. Emollients should be applied regularly through the day and copiously at night, when cotton gloves worn over the top will increase efficacy. Small studies have demonstrated clinical improvement in HFS with the administration of pyridoxine and oral steroid therapy, but there has been no confirmation of these findings in randomized controlled trials to support their widespread use.[5]

What are the other common cutaneous side effects of chemotherapy?
Chemotherapy agents generally target rapidly dividing cells, as a consequence of which they are particularly toxic to organ systems such as skin, nails, hair and the gastrointestinal mucosa. Subsequently, there are wide and varied reports of cutaneous reactions to chemotherapy, an extensive coverage of which is beyond the scope of this chapter.

Hyperpigmentation of the skin, mucous membranes and nails is a common reaction to chemotherapy. Ant-tumour antibiotics, alkylating agents and the fluoropyrimidines are among the commoner drugs to cause hyperpigmentation, which usually affects the skin in a diffuse manner. Local changes may also be seen, and a distinctive supravenous hyperpigmentation caused by fluorouracil and vinorelbine descriptively termed 'serpentine' hyperpigmentation.[6]

Radiation enhancement is an effect of some systemic anticancer treatments whereby the dermatological toxicity of radiotherapy is increased, ranging from a mild rash to severe skin necrosis. Methotrexate, fluorouracil, docetaxel and the anthracyclines are among the drugs implicated. Adjuvant anthracycline treatment is not given alongside adjuvant radiotherapy in the treatment of breast cancer for this very reason.

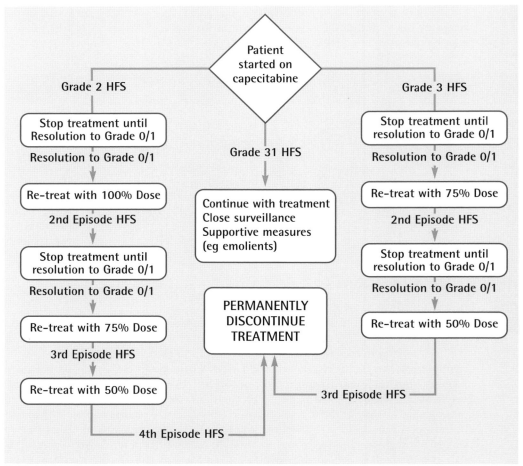

Figure 21.1 Dose management of capecitabine in grade 2/3 HFS.

Additionally, a phenomenon known as radiation recall is sometimes seen, in which areas previously treated with radiotherapy develop an inflammatory skin reaction following administration of chemotherapy. The interval between radiotherapy and radiation recall induced by chemotherapy varies widely, with intravenous drugs usually causing a reaction within minutes to days, whereas the time taken for oral agents usually ranges from days to months.[7]

Typical cutaneous toxicity to tyrosine kinase inhibitors such as erlotinib, gefitinib and sorafenib, includes acneiform (papulopustular) rashes. These can usually be managed with emollients and topical steroid creams, but may require topical antibiotic cream or oral antibiotic therapy, such as tetracyclines as used in acne vulgaris.[8]

Immune-mediated hypersensitivity reactions are seen with many chemotherapy agents. Hypersensitivity reactions to platinum compounds are usually acquired, whereas reactions to taxanes and monoclonal antibodies are commonly immediate and tend to occur within minutes of starting an infusion. Most infusion reactions are Type I hypersensitivity IgE-mediated allergic reactions with urticaria, pruritis, angio-oedema, and other symptoms of anaphylaxis. Type III hypersensitivity reactions may be responsible for erythema multiforme and cutaneous vasculitis, which may be seen secondary to methotrexate and rituximab reactions. Treatment is centred on prevention, with pemetrexed and the taxanes being administered alongside preventative corticosteroids and antihistamines. Treatment of anaphylaxis is exactly as for any other cause and, depending upon the severity of the reaction, may include adrenaline (epinephrine), corticosteroids and antihistamines.

Conclusions

The skin is an organ with vital physiological functions, whose deterioration can cause significant morbidity (both physical and psychological) and, occasionally, mortality. As the number of new chemotherapy agents increases so does the number of cutaneous toxicities. It is important to consider the numerous differential diagnoses for a rash in a cancer patient: cutaneous reaction to another drug, exacerbation of a pre-existing condition, subcutaneous metastases, paraneoplastic phenomenon, photosensitivity, graft-versus-host disease, a nutritional disorder, or a combination of the above. A vigilant, pre-emptive approach with a view to preventing the more severe toxicities is advisable.

Further Reading

1   Cohen PR. Acral erythema: a clinical review. *Cutis* 1993; **51**:175–9.

2   Lacouture ME, Reilly LM, Gerami P, Guitart J. Hand foot skin reaction in cancer patients treated with the multikinase inhibitors sorafenib and sunitinib. *Ann Oncol* 2008; **19**: 1955–61.

3   National Institutes of Health, National Cancer Institute. *Common Terminology Criteria for Adverse Events, version 4.03.* NIH publication no.09-5410 [revised Jun 2010]. Bethesda: National Institutes of Health; 14 Jun 2010.

4   Lassere Y, Hoff P. Management of hand-foot syndrome in patients treated with capecitabine (Xeloda). *Eur J Oncol Nurs* 2004; **8**: S31–S40.

5   Kang YK, Lee SS, Yoon DH, *et al.* Pyridoxine is not effective to prevent hand-foot syndrome associated with capecitabine therapy: results of a randomized, double-blind, placebo-controlled study. *J Clin Oncol* 2010; **28**: 3824–9.

6   Payne AS, James WD, Weiss RB. Dermatologic toxicity of chemotherapeutic agents. *Semin Oncol* 2006; **33**: 86–97.

7   Payne AS, Savarese DMF. *Cutaneous complications of conventional chemotherapy agents* [Internet]. Waltham, Mass.: UpToDate; c.2011–13. Available from: www.uptodate.com/contents/cutaneous-complications-of-conventional-chemotherapy-agents

8   Jacot W, Bessis D, Jorda E, *et al.* Acneiform eruption induced by epidermal growth factor receptor inhibitors in patients with solid tumours. *Br J Dermatol* 2004; **151**: 238–41.

See also:

Ailor SK, Miles SC. Dermatologic Toxicity. In: Perry MC, editor. *The Chemotherapy Source Book.* 4th ed. Philadelphia: Lippincott Williams & Wilkins; 2008. p.136–47.

Hood AF, Haynes HA. Dermatologic complications. In: Holland JF, et al. (editors). *Cancer Medicine.* 4th ed. Baltimore: Williams & Wilkins; 1997. Vol II: p.3141.

PROBLEM

22 Gut Infections and Acute Diarrhoea

Daniel Lee, Alan Anthoney

Case History

A 76-year-old man presents with abdominal pain and diarrhoea. He has metastatic rectal cancer and commenced palliative chemotherapy five weeks ago. He is now on cycle 2 day 16 of oxaliplatin and capecitabine.

The patient's stool has been loose and watery for two days; he has been opening his bowels six times a day and had some incontinence. He stopped his capecitabine tablets on the day of admission on the advice of the oncology unit.

On examination the patient appeared fatigued and dehydrated. His pulse was 110 bpm and his blood pressure 105/65 mmHg; his temperature was 36.9°C. Heart sounds were normal. He had a tender abdomen and bowel sounds were present; there was no guarding or rebound.

The patient was placed in a side room and stool samples were taken. Intravenous fluids were initiated and he was commenced on loperamide tablets. The patient's chemotherapy was withheld.

What are the potential causes of diarrhoea in this patient?

How would you manage diarrhoea in a patient such as this?

What recent developments are there in the management of diarrhoea in this group of patients?

What other GI tract toxicity can occur due to anticancer therapy?

Background

Diarrhoea is a common side effect of systemic therapy and can affect up to 80% of patients depending on the regimen. It can manifest as a low-grade but persistent annoyance, up to a life-threatening toxicity requiring inpatient admission and urgent medical care.

What are the potential causes of diarrhoea in this patient?

It is important to distinguish between the differing aetiologies for diarrhoea in a patient such as this who is receiving treatment for cancer. In such patients, aetiologies include chemotherapy, infection or radiotherapy. Of particular note is that there may have been a disturbed gastrointestinal (GI) tract from previous surgery in this patient. This may result in altered gastric emptying, altered bile salt flow, bacterial overgrowth, or hepatic insufficiency; these all result in diarrhoea, which may be exacerbated by systemic anticancer treatment. Radiotherapy, abdominal surgery or the cancer itself can lead to bowel obstruction with associated overflow diarrhoea. Areas particularly prone to obstruction include the small bowel and the sigmoid colon after pelvic radiotherapy.

How would you manage diarrhoea in a patient such as this?

The management of cancer patients receiving systemic therapy who develop diarrhoea can be markedly different from that on a general medical ward, as antidiarrhoeals may need to be used early and aggressively before the results of stool cultures are obtained. A common assessment and treatment pathway for patients with diarrhoea on chemotherapy is outlined in Figure 22.1.

Gut Infection

Cytotoxic chemotherapy agents directly affect the gastrointestinal mucosa and cause inflammation, oedema, ulceration and atrophy. This leads to increased permeability of the bowel mucosa and increased susceptibility to transmural infection. This can lead to septicaemia and shock, especially if it coincides with neutropenia from the chemotherapy.

The GI symptoms caused through infection can respond quickly to antibiotics. The work-up of such patients should be timely, as appropriate early intervention can reduce morbidity and mortality. Organisms leading to infection include *Clostridium difficile*, coliforms, fungal infections and viruses.

Clostridium difficile is the most commonly associated pathogen, and may not be associated with prior antibiotic use in patients on chemotherapy. The diarrhoea is toxin-mediated, and this is important in the detection of active disease. Colonoscopy is not usually clinically indicated but demonstrates typical yellow pseudomembranes. Any causative antibiotics should be stopped and chemotherapy should be withheld. Treatment includes oral metronidazole or vancomycin depending on local protocol and severity. In cases associated with toxic megacolon a senior oncological and senior surgical review should be undertaken urgently.

Acute diarrhoea secondary to anticancer treatment

Chemotherapy-induced diarrhoea (CID) can occur in up to 80% of patients, depending on the chemotherapy regimen. Table 22.1 provides a summary of commonly used chemotherapy regimens in colorectal cancer.

There are multiple considerations for those with CID, some of the more commonly encountered scenarios are detailed below.

1. Oral anticancer treatments

Orally administered treatments that are associated with diarrhoea are of particular importance. Some patients, in the hope of increasing treatment effectiveness, will continue to take their tablets in spite of severe toxicity. Good patient selection and education can reduce the morbidity associated with this treatment route.

Figure 22.1 Management diagram for patients with diarrhoea on chemotherapy

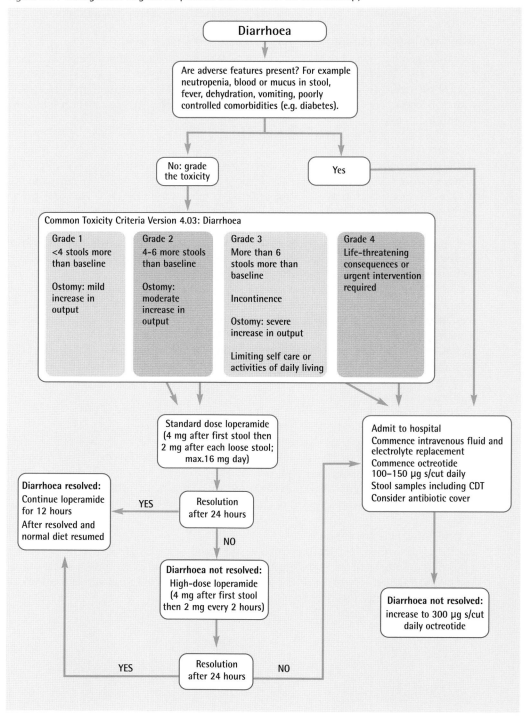

Table 22.1 Chemotherapy regimens and average rates of severe diarrhoea	
Chemotherapy regimen	Diarrhoea – grade 3/4
5-FU (bolus)	32%
Irinotecan	20%
Capecitabine	10–15%
Docetaxel	
100 mg/m^2	4%
75 mg/m^2	1.7%
FOLFOX	8.6%
FOLFIRI	24%
FOLFOX + Bevacizumab	13.2%

5-FU, fluorouracil; FOLFOX, leuovorin + 5-FU + oxaliplatin; FOLFIRI, leuovorin + 5-FU + irinotecan

2. Fluorouracil (5-FU) and dihydropyrimidine dehydrogenase (DPYD)

Up to 5% of patients are deficient in DPYD, which is an enzyme central to fluorouracil catabolism. In these cases, diarrhoea and other toxicities can occur early and be particularly severe. Patients should be managed aggressively as described above, and further fluorouracil use would not be recommended.

3. Irinotecan

Irinotecan is associated with two distinct forms of diarrhoea. Early-onset diarrhoea is associated with an acute cholinergic reaction and is often seen with rhinitis and salivation. This should be treated with atropine and will usually resolve quickly. Late-onset diarrhoea is particularly difficult; it is associated with the metabolism of irinotecan metabolites within the GI tract and can produce profuse diarrhoea. It occurs from days 7 to 10, corresponding with neutropenia. Ciprofloxacin is often used to cover for gram-negative sepsis.

4. Biological treatment

Diarrhoea is a common side effect of biological therapies (or biologics) and can occur in up to 60% of patients. The severity of diarrhoea is dependent on both the drug and its combination with other biological agents or chemotherapies. Particularly important biological anticancer agents commonly used are listed in Table 22.2.

Ipilimumab affects the body's immune response to cancer cells by modulating the T-cell immune system. It can be associated with diarrhoea, and if grade ≥3, steroids may be indicated. This is potentially life-threatening and should be treated in accordance with local protocols.

Table 22.2 Rates of diarrhoea in commonly used biological anticancer agents

Drug	Diarrhoea Any grade	Diarrhoea Grade 3/4	Special consideration
Erlotinib (NSCLC)	54%	6%	
Lapatinib in combination with capecitabine (1000 mg/m²)	65%	Rare	Responds quickly to antidiarrhoeals
Sunitinib	52.3%	5.9%	
Bevacizumab	21%	1%	Low association with gastrointestinal fistulae and perforation
Ipilimumab	20%	4.5%	Occasionally fatal – refer to protocol for dose delay and adjuvants

5. Chemo-radiotherapy

Patients receiving concurrent chemotherapy and radiotherapy may be more susceptible to diarrhoea, particular if receiving radiotherapy treatment to the pelvic region. The peak incidence is one to two weeks after radiotherapy, when the toxicity to the GI mucosa is at its highest.

6. Neutropenia and typhlitis

Typhlitis is bowel inflammation usually involving the caecum in a patient with chemotherapy-induced neutropenia. It is associated with a triad of right lower quadrant pain, fever and bloody diarrhoea. The patient should receive treatment like any other neutropenic patient alongside aggressive antidiarrhoea management. There is a high mortality associated with this rare condition. If the bleeding is severe, surgical intervention may be necessary if clinically appropriate.

7. Adjuvants to treatment

Supportive medications alongside systemic treatment can also lead to diarrhoea. These include antibiotics, antiemetics, laxatives and some herbal remedies. These should be considered alongside a general medical and medicine review.

What recent developments are there in the management of diarrhoea in this group of patients?

Prophylaxis

Multiple trials have tried to identify the optimum prophylactic measure for CID. Probiotics have produced mixed results in diarrhoea of all causes, but needs further large trials in the chemotherapy-receiving population. Budesonide can reduce the gastrointestinal mucosal inflammation in association with chemotherapy but needs further study. Long-acting octreotide has been used, without clinical trial, for rectal cancer patients at high risk of CID, and in those with severe diarrhoea but in whom dose reduction is not desirable.

Enzyme deficiency assays

There are multiple commercial assays available or under development attempting to predict the likelihood of severe diarrhoea prior to commencing chemotherapy, e.g. DPYD for 5-FU use and UGT for irinotecan. Current limitations are the number of possible mutation sites and trying to identify the most common and clinically significant of these.

Clostridium difficile *toxin assay*

Assays for *C. difficile* toxin are under development to expedite diagnosis and therefore management.

What other gastrointestinal tract toxicity can occur due to anticancer therapy?

The main other GI toxicity that occurs as a result of anticancer treatment with either chemotherapy, radiotherapy or a combination of both, is mucositis. Mucositis is inflammation and ulceration of the mucous membranes lining the GI tract. It can occur anywhere along the GI tract, most commonly in the mouth, and is a common and often debilitating complication of treatment that can lead to the need for acute admission for treatment. Mucositis affects almost all patients undergoing intensive and high-dose chemotherapy and haematopoietic stem cell transplantation, and patients receiving radiotherapy for head and neck cancers, but also affects a wide range of other patients receiving chemotherapy to varying degrees. Overall, between 5%–15% of patients get mucositis while receiving anticancer treatment.

The severity of oral mucositis can be evaluated using appropriate assessment tools, such as the Common Terminology Criteria for Adverse Events (CTCAE) version 4 and graded from 0–4 as seen in Table 22.3.

Table 22.3 Common Terminology Criteria for Adverse Events (CTCAE) grading for oral mucositis	
0	None
1	Painless ulcers, erythema, or mild soreness in the absence of lesions
2	Painful erythema, oedema or ulcers but can eat or swallow
3	Painful erythema, oedema or ulcers requiring IV hydration
4	Severe ulceration or requires parenteral or enteral nutritional support or prophylactic intubation

The management of oral mucositis is largely supportive, with promotion of good oral hygiene being vital when trying to avoid superadded infection. Mouthwashes with anaesthetic can help to relieve pain, as can barrier protection agents such as Gelclair. Adequate hydration in patients unable to swallow or eat is important, and in the event of prolonged mucositis it may sometimes be necessary to consider parenteral or enteral nutrition.

Conclusion

Diarrhoea is a common and important toxicity. Its management in cancer patients differs from that in other medical specialties and the early and aggressive use of antidiarrhoeals is paramount. Good patient education and support can reduce the morbidity, and efficient clinician response can reduce its mortality further.

Further Reading

Andreyev HJV, Davidson SE, Gillespie C, *et al.* Practice guidance on the management of acute and chronic gastrointestinal problems arising as a result of treatment for cancer. *Gut* 2012; **61**: 179–92.

Maroun JA, Anthony LB, Blais N, *et al.* Prevention and management of chemotherapy-induced diarrhoea in patients with colorectal cancer: a consensus statement by the Canadian Working Group on Chemotherapy-Induced Diarrhoea. *Curr Oncol* 2007; **14**(1): 13–20

Stein A, Voigt W, Jordan K. Chemotherapy-induced diarrhoea: pathophysiology, frequency and guideline-based management. *Ther Adv Med Oncol* 2010; **2**(1): 51–63.

23 Peripheral Neurotoxicity

Greg Heath, Susan Short, Helen Ford

Case History

A 65-year-old man with colorectal cancer presents to clinic to receive the results of his restaging scan following six cycles of oxaliplatin and fluorouracil (5-FU) 'modified de Gramont' (MdG) chemotherapy regime. He complains of shooting pains in his hands when he touches cold objects, and difficulty in performing fine motor tasks such as buttoning his shirt because his hands feel like 'cotton wool'.

What is the most likely diagnosis?

What are the risk factors for this complication?

What are the treatment options?

Background

What is the most likely diagnosis?

This patient is suffering from a grade 3 oxaliplatin-induced peripheral neuropathy (see Table 23.1).

Table 23.1	National Institute of Cancer Common Toxic Criteria (NIC-CTC) for sensory neuropathy
Grade 0	Normal
Grade 1	Loss of deep tendon reflexes or paraesthesia not interfering with function
Grade 2	Objective sensory loss or paraesthesia interfering with function but not with activities of daily living
Grade 3	Sensory loss or paraesthesia interfering with activities of daily living
Grade 4	Permanent sensory loss that interferes with function

Oxaliplatin, a third-generation platinum compound, is associated with two forms of peripheral neuropathy: the first, an acute neurosensory complex, occurs either during or immediately after receiving the infusion; and the second, a cumulative sensory neuropathy (represented by the case above) which appears to be dose-limiting and later in onset.

Acute neurological symptoms are common with oxaliplatin. Indeed, in their prospective study, Argyriou *et al.* noted neurological symptoms in 86% of their 170 patient cohort.[1] Of these, cold-induced perioral paraesthesia and cold-induced pharyngolaryngeal dysaesthesia were the most frequent symptoms experienced. Other symptoms included jaw stiffness, dysphagia and muscle cramps.

Neurophysiologically, cumulative sensory neuropathy is the result of axonal damage to the large, myelinated nerve fibres. Both oxaliplatin and its more neurotoxic counterpart, cisplatin, enter the dorsal root ganglion and bind to nuclear and mitochondrial DNA, thereby causing apoptosis. Cisplatin appears to be more neurotoxic than oxaliplatin owing to its greater propensity to form platinum–DNA adducts.[2] Other chemotherapy agents associated with peripheral neuropathy are illustrated in Table 23.2.

Table 23.2 Chemotherapy agents associated with peripheral neuropathy

Agent	Oncological uses	Neurological complications
Paclitaxel	Ovarian, breast, lung, head and neck cancers	Motor neuropathy (proximal muscle weakness), acute myalgia, sensory neuropathy
Docetaxel	Non-small cell lung, breast and ovarian cancers	Motor neuropathy, sensory neuropathy, less severe than paclitaxel
Thalidomide	Multiple myeloma	Sensory neuropathy
Bortezomib	Multiple myeloma	Sensory neuropathy
Vincristine	Non-Hodgkin lymphoma, leukaemia	Sensory>motor neuropathy, autonomic neuropathy

What are the risk factors for this complication?

The likelihood of experiencing acute symptoms with oxaliplatin is greater with doses ≥ 130 mg/m^2 than at ≤ 85 mg/m^2 and is dependent on the infusion rate.[3] Reducing the infusion rate from 2 to 6 hours may ameliorate the symptoms and reduce the risk of recurrence.

The risk of developing late-onset peripheral neuropathy is correlated positively with the cumulative dose of oxaliplatin. In a literature review, the incidence of neuropathy was 10% and 15% with cumulative doses of 780 and 850 mg/m^2, respectively.[4] Patients who develop complex acute neurological symptoms seem also to be at risk of developing severe cumulative neurotoxicity. Although there is a paucity of other risk factors documented in the literature,[5] clinicians should be vigilant in identifying patients with a pre-existing neuropathy before commencing chemotherapy. One group of patients for whom this may be particularly relevant are those with diabetes mellitus. A full sensory examination should be conducted beforehand, with avoidance of neurotoxic agents if there is evidence of neuropathy.

Investigators with an interest in pharmacogenetics have explored polymorphisms that may influence the risk of developing platinum-based neurotoxicity. One study has revealed that polymorphism to the drug-metabolising enzyme glutathione S-transferase was more common in those patients suffering from grade 3 neurotoxicity having been administered oxaliplatin.[6] Notwithstanding, future studies are warranted before pharmacogenetic profiling can be justified.

What are the treatment options?

In the majority of cases, oxaliplatin-induced peripheral neuropathy is reversible. In the MOSAIC trial, in which patients were randomized to receive adjuvant chemotherapy in the form of 5-FU plus leuovorin with and without oxaliplatin ($85\,mg/m^2$ every two weeks) over 24 weeks, 13% of patients receiving oxaliplatin developed grade 3 toxicity, which reduced to 0.7% by 48 months.[7] Thus, if the oxaliplatin treatment is stopped, there is a significant chance that the patient's neuropathy will resolve over time.

In contrast to its less toxic counterpart, the neuropathy associated with cisplatin may continue to progress even on discontinuation of treatment.[8] Moreover, in cisplatin-treated survivors of testicular cancer, the severity of neurotoxicity appears to correlate positively to the level of residual serum platinum.[9] Although increasing the infusion time may assuage acute neurological symptoms, such a strategy has not proved to be as beneficial in combating the signs and symptoms associated with cumulative toxicity.[10]

A protective effect of vitamin E has been conjectured by investigators. The largest placebo-controlled randomized trial, which analysed 41 patients (17 receiving vitamin E and 24 receiving placebo) who had received at least $300\ mg/m^2$ of cisplatin, demonstrated a lower incidence of grade 3 neurotoxicity in the vitamin E arm.[11] Those receiving vitamin E were administered a dose of 400 IU daily during treatment and for three months following discontinuation of treatment. Owing to the fact that administration of vitamin E does not have a deleterious effect on antitumour activity, it may be reasonable to recommend this treatment in patients expecting to receive a dose exceeding $300\ mg/m^2$. That said, larger, randomized controlled trials are needed before this approach is adopted universally.

Numerous agents have been purported to be beneficial in ameliorating peripheral neurological symptoms associated with platinum-based chemotherapy, including amifostine and glutathione.[12,13] However, a Cochrane Database review suggested that there is insufficient evidence to support the use of such agents.[14] There are two notable caveats to this review: it did not review the role of intravenous magnesium or calcium infusions, nor the effects of the antidepressant venlafaxine.

Venlafaxine has been investigated in one small, placebo-controlled, randomized trial.[15] Patients were randomly assigned to receive 50 mg venlafaxine one hour prior to the infusion and 37.5 mg twice daily from days 2 to 11. Not only did the venlafaxine group experience fewer acute symptoms, the percentage of those experiencing no neurotoxicity after three months post-treatment in the venlafaxine group compared to the placebo group was 39% and 6%, respectively. Although randomized studies are warranted before the use of this drug can be recommended, the results from the aforementioned trial are promising.

Two phase III placebo-controlled trials aimed to explore the merits of administering intravenous calcium and magnesium prior to delivery of oxaliplatin in patients treated for colorectal cancer, one in the adjuvant setting (NCCTG N04C7) and one in the palliative setting (CONcePT).[16,17] In the double-blind, placebo-controlled NCCTG N04C7 trial, the calcium and magnesium infusion appeared to reduce the severity and delay the time to acquire neurotoxicity. Disappointingly, the effects on tumour growth could not be analysed due to unsubstantiated concerns that it may adversely affect such oncological outcomes.[16] An interim analysis report of the CONcePT trial demonstrated a lower tumour response rate in those patients receiving magnesium and calcium infusions and, although an independent blinded central review of the response data from this trial subsequently did not support this, the study was discontinued early.[17]

The intention of the CAIRO2 trial (NCT00208546) was to compare capecitabine, oxaliplatin and bevacizumab with or without cetuximab in previously untreated patients with metastatic colorectal cancer.[18] Physicians introduced intravenous magnesium and calcium at their own discretion. The results are noteworthy because no differences in tumour response rates were noted between those receiving the electrolyte infusion and those receiving the chemotherapy alone. Moreover, the incidence of all grades of late neurotoxicity was less in the magnesium/calcium infusion group.

In summary, it appears that calcium and magnesium infusions may be useful in patients treated for metastatic disease. Further studies are warranted to explore the safety of this regimen in the adjuvant setting.

Drugs aimed at addressing neuropathic pain, for example pregabalin or gabapentin, may be employed to assuage the pain associated with chemotherapy-induced peripheral neuropathy. The use of such agents is discussed in another case study (Chapter 44, *see* p.227) and will not be elaborated further here.

Conclusion

Peripheral neuropathy is a common complication of platinum chemotherapy and may be irreversible. Although new treatments are under investigation, the use of intravenous magnesium and calcium in patients treated for metastatic disease may reduce the severity of neuropathy.

Further reading

1   Argyriou AA, Cavaletti G, Briani C, *et al*. Clinical pattern and associations of oxaliplatin acute neurotoxicity: A prospective study in 170 patients with colorectal cancer. *Cancer* 2013; **119**(2): 438–44.

2   Ta LE, Espeset L, Podtratz J, Windebank AJ. Neurotoxicity of oxaliplatin and cisplatin for dorsal root ganglion neurons correlates with platinum-DNA binding. *Neurotoxicology* 2006; **27**(6): 992–1002.

3   Gamelin E, Gamelin L, Bosi L, Quasthoff S. Clinical aspects and molecular basis of oxaliplatin neurotoxicity: current management and development of preventive measures. *Semin Oncol* 2002; **29**: 21–33.

4   Cassidy J, Misset JL. Oxaliplatin-related side effects: characteristics and management. *Semin Oncol* 2002; **29**: 11–20.

5   Alejandro LM, Behrendt CE, Chen K, Openshaw H, Shibata S. Predicting acute and persisting neuropathy associated with oxaliplatin. *Am J Clin Oncol* 2012; **36**(4): 331–7.

6   Ruzzo A, Graziano F, Loupakis F, *et al*. Pharmacogenetic profiling in patients with advanced colorectal cancer treated with first-line FOLFOX-4 chemotherapy. *J Clin Oncol* 2007; **25**(10): 1247–54.

7   Andre T, Boni C, Navarro M, *et al*. Improved overall survival with oxaliplatin, fluorouracil, and leucovorin as adjuvant treatment in stage II or III colon cancer in the MOSAIC trial. *J Clin Oncol* 2009; **27**(19): 3109–16.

8   Von Schlippe M, Fowler CJ, Harland SJ. Cisplatin neurotoxicity in the treatment of metastatic germ cell tumour: time course and prognosis. *Br J Cancer* 2001; **85**(6); 823–6.

9   Sprauten M, Darrah, TH, Peterson DR, *et al.* Impact of long term serum platinum concentrations on neuro- and ototoxicity in cisplatin treated survivors of testicular cancer. *J Clin Oncol* 2012; **30**(3): 300–7.

10 Petrioli R, Pascucci A, Francinic E, *et al.* Neurotoxicity of FOLFOX-4 as adjuvant treatment for patients with colon and gastric cancer: a randomized study of two different schedules of oxaliplatin. *Cancer Chemother Pharmacol* 2008; **61**(1): 105–11.

11 Pace A, Giannarelli D, Galie E, *et al.* Vitamin E neuroprotection for cisplatin neuropathy: a randomized, placebo- controlled trial. *Neurology* 2010; **74**(9): 762–6.

12 Moore DH, Donnelly J, McGuire WP, *et al.* Limited access trial using amifostine for protection against cisplatin- and three- hour paclitaxel – induced neurotoxicity: a phase II study of the Gynecologic Oncology Group. *J Clin Onol* 2003; **21**(22): 4207–13.

13 Cascinu S, Catalano V, Cordella L, *et al.* Neuroprotective effect of reduced glutathione on oxaliplatin – based chemotherapy in advanced colorectal cancer: a randomized, double-blind, placebo-controlled trial. *J Clin Oncol* 2002; **20**(16); 3478–83.

14 Albers JW, Chaudhry V, Cavaletti G, Donehower RC. Interventions for preventing neuropathy caused by cisplatin and related compounds. Cochrane Database Syst Rev 2011; (2): CD005228.

15 Durand JP, Deplanque G, Montheil V, *et al.* Efficacy of venlafaxine for the prevention and relief of oxaliplain-induced acute neurotoxicity: results of EFFOX, a randomized, double-blind, placebo controlled phase III trial. *Ann Oncol* 2012; **23**(1): 200–5.

16 Grothey A, Nikcevich DA, Sloan JA, *et al.* Intravenous calcium and magnesium for oxaliplatin – induced sensory neurotoxicity in adjuvant colon cancer: NCCTG N04C7. *J Clin Oncol* 2011; **29**(4): 421–7.

17 Grothey A, Hart LL, Rowland KM, *et al.* Intermittent oxliplatin administraton and time to treatment failure in metastatic colorectal cancer: Final results of the phase III CONcePT trial. *J Clin Oncol* 2008; **26**(suppl): abstract 4010.

18 Knijn N, Tol J, Koopman M, *et al.* The effect of prophylactic calcium and magnesium infusions on the incidence of neurotoxicity and clinical outcome of oxaliplatin-based systemic treatment in advanced colorectal cancer patients. *Eur J Cancer* 2011; **47**(3): 369–74.

PROBLEM

24 Central Neurotoxicity

Greg Heath, Susan Short, Helen Ford

Case History

A 55-year-old man administering sunitinib for one week for metastatic renal cell carcinoma is admitted onto the acute oncology ward with a 24-hour history of increasing confusion, blurred vision and generalized headaches which appeared to come on suddenly. On examination his Glasgow Coma Scale (GCS) score is 14/15 (due to confusion). Visual acuities are 6/36 bilaterally. His pupil reactions are normal and his ocular fundi appears normal. His blood pressure is 160/110 mmHg (previously normotensive). There is no meningism and no other neurological abnormalities can be detected.

What is your differential diagnosis?

How would you investigate this patient?

What is the most likely diagnosis and its pathogenesis?

What is the prognosis and management?

Background

What is your differential diagnosis?

The causes for an altered mental status are legion. Broad neurological categories to consider include vascular events (haemorrhage, ischaemia/infarction), space-occupying lesions causing mass effect, and infection. In the context of a patient undergoing chemotherapy one must also consider CNS side-effects related to the drug. The differential diagnoses may include the following:

Unrelated to the drug

• Brain metastases

• Haemorrhage or infarct

Drug related

• Posterior reversible encephalopathy syndrome (PRES)

• Infection.

How would you investigate this patient?

Neuroimaging plays an essential role in investigating patients with acute cognitive decline and positive abnormal neurological signs. In the first instance, computed tomography

(CT) imaging of the patient's head is quick to perform and may identify haemorrhage, brain metastases and infarcts. Magentic resonance imaging (MRI) should be performed if the images acquired by CT are equivocal. The patient's T2-weighted MRI scans revealed hyperintense lesions predominantly in the parietal areas, together with some occipital involvement (see Figures 24.1A and B).

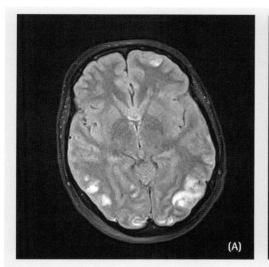
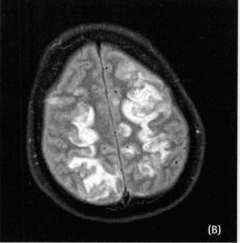

Figure 24.1 Hyperintense lesions involving parieto-occipital junction (A). Hyperintense lesions within parietal lobes (B).

What is the most likely diagnosis and its pathogenesis?

The MRI findings, hypertension, visual symptoms and headaches with sudden onset following the introduction of chemotherapy suggest a diagnosis of PRES secondary to sunitinib. The terms reversible posterior leukoencephalopathy syndrome and reversible posterior cerebral oedema syndrome are interchangeable with PRES.

Drugs attributed to this disorder include immunosuppressive agents such as ciclosporin and tacrolimus, and typically occur within two weeks of commencing these agents.[1,2] It is noteworthy that the drug serum levels tend to be within the therapeutic range.[1]

Numerous chemotherapeutic agents have been associated with this disorder, including gemcitabine, cytarabine, cisplatin and bevacizumab.[1,3,4]

The pathogenesis of PRES is poorly understood. Notwithstanding, there are two theories: the first and most popular theory relates to the breakdown of cerebral autoregulation following a rapid rise in blood pressure, resulting in breakdown of the blood-brain barrier;[5] the second suggests that endothelial dysfunction attributed to circulating toxins may alter the blood–brain barrier, leading to extravasation.[6] This second theory may be particularly pertinent to chemotherapy and immunosuppressive agents, since patients diagnosed with PRES while being administered the latter often have lower average pressures than other PRES sufferers.[2]

Albeit rare, there is an increasing number of case reports within the medical literature of patients acquiring PRES secondary to sunitinib.[7] Sunitinib is a multi targeted tyrosine kinase inhibitor that inhibits the vascular endothelial growth factor (VEGF) receptor and platelet-derived growth factor (PDGF) receptor. It is noteworthy that in nearly half of the reported cases, hypertension is present at diagnosis,[8] and the onset of symptoms after commencing the drug range from one week to eight months.[7]

What is the prognosis and management?

As its name suggests, PRES is often reversible. Indeed, in the review of cases caused by sunitinib, all resolved over time. In a study cohort of 25 patients with PRES due to various causes, Roth and Ferbert noted three to have a poor outcome.[9] Morbidity was associated with either concomitant sepsis or intracerebral haemorrhage in such cases.

Symptomatic and radiological resolution of signs are not contemporaneous. Typically, the former resolve within 3–8 days whereas the latter take longer.[9] Repeat MRI scanning is recommended approximately 10 days after the onset of symptoms, when either total resolution or at least diminution of signs should be present.

Management is not evidence based, but the principles are as follows: first, remove the inciting agent; second, control hypertension and fluid balance; and third, control of seizures (if present) using antiepileptic medication.

In the absence of hypertension and seizures, removal of the offending agent, together with close monitoring of fluid balance and blood pressure, may be all that is required. Control of hypertension may need to be done in a hig-dependency setting with close blood pressure monitoring, especially if the patient is suffering from seizures or a fluctuating GCS. The use of intravenous agents, such as labetalol, is highly recommended in such circumstances. Alternatively treatment with oral agents such as nimodipine modified release will suffice.

Intravenous phenytoin may be used in patients who are in status epilepticus or are developing frequent seizures. Other antiepileptic drugs, such as levetiracetam, can also be incorporated into the patient's treatment regimen. The seizures associated with PRES rarely persist and antiepileptic medication may be withdrawn within three months of commencing treatment.[1,9]

Conclusion

Although a relatively rare phenomenon, more people are acquiring PRES as a result of the increase in the oncologist's therapeutic armamentarium. Practitioners should immediately consider this diagnosis in anybody presenting with visual disturbance, headaches and/or seizures, especially patients who have recently commenced chemotherapy, since early treatment leads to abrogation of the signs and symptoms.

Further reading

1 Roth C, Ferbert A. The posterior reversible encephalopathy syndrome: what's certain, what's new? *Pract Neurol* 2011; **11**: 136–44.

2 Burnett MM, Hess CP, Roberts JP, *et al*. Presentation of reversible posterior leukoencephalopathy syndrome in patients on calcineurin inhibitors. *Clin Neurol Neurosurg* 2010; **112**: 886–91.

3 Ito Y, Arahata Y, Goto Y, *et al*. Cisplatin neurotoxicity presenting as reversible posterior leukoencephalopathy syndrome. *Am J Neuroradiol* 1998; **19**(3): 415–7.

4 Ozcan C, Wong SJ, Hari P. Reversible posterior leukoencephalopathy syndrome and bevacizumab. *N Engl J Med* 2006; **354**(9): 980–-2.

5 Schwartz RB, Jones KM, Kalina P, *et al*. Hypertensive encephalopathy: findings on CT, MR imaging, and SPECT imaging in 14 cases. *Am J Roentgenol* 1992; **159**: 379–83.

6 Bartynski WS, Boardman JF, Zeigler ZR,et al. Posterior reversible encephalopathy syndrome in infection, sepsis and shock. *Am J Neuroradiol* 2006; **27**: 2179–90.

7 Padhy BM, Shanmugam SP, Gupta YK, Goyal A. Reversible posterior leukoencephalopathy syndrome in an elderly male on sunitinib therapy. *Br J Clin Pharmacol* 2011; **71**(5): 777–9.

8 Chen A, Agarwal N. Reversible posterior leucoencephalopathy syndrome associated with sunitinib. *Int Med J* 2009; **39**: 341–2.

9 Roth C, Ferbert A. posterior reversible encephalopathy syndrome: long term follow-up. *J Neurol Neurosurg Psychiatry* 2010; **81**: 773–7.

Acknowledgements

The authors would like to thank Dr Ian Craven, Consultant Neuroradiologist at Leeds Teaching Hospital NHS Trust for providing the images in Figure 24.1.

25 Chemotherapy-Induced Lung Toxicity

Lisa Owen, Satiavani Ramasamy, Dan Stark, Paul Plant

Case History

A 48-year-old man finished his forth BEP (bleomycin/etoposide/cisplatin) cycle for stage IV non-seminomatous germ cell tumour four weeks ago. He now presents with a four-day history of increasing shortness of breath and a dry cough.

On examination, the patient had the following:temperature 37.9°C; SpO$_2$ on air, 90%; respiratory rate, 22 breaths per minute. Chest examination revealed fine bibasal crackles.

What are the differential diagnoses?

What investigations do you require?

How would you manage this patient?

Background

What are the differential diagnoses?

It is not an uncommon event for patients who are receiving, or who have previously received, systemic oncological treatment to present with respiratory symptoms. Depending on other associated symptoms and timing in relation to treatment, the spectrum of respiratory pathologies include:

- Metastases/disease progression
- Infection – typical and atypical
- Pulmonary embolus
- Drug induced
- Pneumonitis
- Idiosyncratic e.g. methotrexate
- Dose related e.g. bleomycin
- Radiation-induced
- Pulmonary oedema
- Cardiogenic
- Non-cardiogenic
- Pulmonary haemorrhage
- Veno-occlusive disease e.g. busulphan.

Infective events are common in patients receiving chemotherapy and can be caused by bacteria, virus or fungi. Neutropenic patients are most at risk, and prolonged periods of neutropenia increase the risk of fungal infections. General debility and hospital stays are additional risk factors.

The following text will discuss chemotherapy-induced lung toxicity in more detail.

Chemotherapy–induced interstitial lung toxicity

Around 10%–20% of patients treated with chemotherapy develop some form of lung toxicity, with over 150 drugs having been implicated.[1] Table 25.1 illustrates the commonest causal agents. With the increasing use of targeted agents and chemo-radiotherapy, we would expect an increase in the incidence.

Bleomycin is one of the most studied agents in the literature in relation to lung toxicity. It has been reported that up to 10% of patients treated with bleomycin develop some pulmonary fibrosis, in 25% of whom it can be fatal. It occurs more frequently in the first six months after treatment, but can occur many years later and is best considered a lifetime risk.[2]

Pathogenesis

The mechanism behind chemotherapy-induced lung toxicity is poorly understood. Most information is known about bleomycin-induced toxicity, which is thought to be predominantly due to free radical damage.[3] Bleomycin hydrolase is responsible for inactivating bleomycin in both normal and tumour tissues, and lack of this enzyme has been implicated in the pathogenesis of lung toxicity. There is an innate low activity of bleomycin hydrolase in the skin and lung, perhaps explaining why these organs are most commonly affected.[3] Several other mechanisms have been suggested in relation to other chemotherapy-induced lung toxicities including:[1,4]

- Direct injury to the pneumocytes resulting in systemic release of cytokines and accumulation of inflammatory cells (e.g. cyclophosphamide).
- Epidermal growth factor receptors (EGFR) are found on type II pneumocytes and are an important factor in repair; hence, agents targeting EGFR may affect tissue repair.
- Radiation recall – subclinical lung damage during radiotherapy that only becomes evident when a further insult to the lung occurs, such as chemotherapy; this is typically described with doxorubicin to actinomycin D, and the cardinal feature is that the pulmonary pathology is tightly delineated to the radiation field.

Risk factors

Risk factors are best studied in relation to bleomycin lung toxicity. In one prospective study the Royal Marsden NHS Trust hospital reported an increased risk with increasing age of the patient (>40 years), poor renal function (GFR <80 ml/min), stage IV disease at presentation, and a cumulative dose of bleomycin >300 000 IU.[5] Renal insufficiency is a risk factor for all renally-excreted drugs.[6] With other chemotherapeutic agents the risk is not always dose dependent, as shown in Table 25.2. The concurrent use of other chemotherapy agents or radiotherapy also has a bearing on the incidence of lung toxicity.[4] Use of high-dose oxygen (which generates free radicals) alongside bleomycin increases the risk of bleomycin lung toxicity and can be a lifelong risk.[4] Other factors, such as underlying lung disease (both benign and malignant) and previous asbestos exposure, have also been implicated in the development of chemotherapy-related lung toxicity.

Table 25.1 List of systemic oncological treatments associated with pneumonitis

Antibiotics	Approximate incidence of lung toxicity
Bleomycin	20%
Mitomycin C	8%
Alkylating agents	
Carmustine (BCNU)	1.5%–20%
Busulfan	6%
Cyclophosphamide	1%
Chlorambucil	<1%
Melphalan	50% asymptomatic histopathological changes
Antimetabolites	
Methotrexate	0%–12% (mortality 1%)
Gemcitabine	0.02%–0.27% (mortality up to 20%)
Fludarabine	8.6%
Podophyllotoxin	
Etoposide	<3%
Taxanes	
Paclitaxel	0.73%–12%
Docetaxel	7%–26%
Targeted agents	
Gefitinib	1%–2% (mortality 33%)
Imatinib	Very rare
Erlotinib	0.8%
Everolimus	8%–14%
Temsirolimus	1%–36%
Topoisomerase I inhibitor	
Irinotecan	1.8%

Presentation

The commonest symptoms include dyspnoea, dry cough, low-grade fever and hypoxaemia. Presentation can be acute or subacute, and onset can range from weeks to years following drug administration. Examination of the chest can be normal or reveal bibasal crackles. Approximately 10% are only identified radiologically.[6] Pneumonitis can be graded as per the Common Terminology Criteria for Adverse Events (CTCAE), shown in Table 25.3.

Table 25.2 Type of renal insufficiency caused by types of chemotherapy drugs

Idiosyncratic	Dose dependent
Methotrexate	Bleomycin
Temsirolimus	Carmustine (BCNU)
Targeted molecules	Busulfan
	Chlorambucil
	Taxanes

What investigations do you require?

The diagnosis that the lung disease is due to chemotherapy is one of exclusion, although there are suggestive biopsy appearances (see Figure 25.1). It is imperative to obtain an accurate drug history. The following tests should be performed:

- Bloods – including full blood count, biochemistry, C-reactive protein, and blood cultures to exclude infective causes
- Arterial blood gas
- Chest X-ray – can be normal or show evidence of unilateral/bilateral reticular shadowing or ground glass opacities

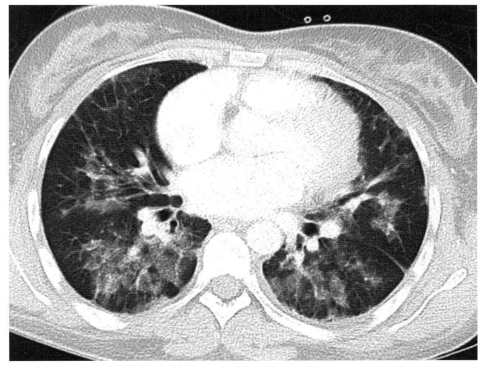

Figure 25.1 Axial slice of CT chest with bleomycin-induced lung toxicity.

- Pulmonary function tests – reveal a restrictive pattern with reduced total lung capacity and reduced forced vital capacity. A reduced diffusing capacity for carbon monoxide can precede clinical and radiographic findings by days to weeks[1]
- High-resolution computerized tomography (HRCT) – common abnormalities are ground glass opacities, consolidation, interlobular septal thickening and nodules[7]
- Bronchoscopy and broncheoalveolar lavage (BAL) – to help exclude infection, haemorrhage and malignancy; samples should be sent for microscopy, sensitivity and culture, alcohol and acid-fast bacilli culture (AAFB), viruses, fungi and cytology.

How would you manage this patient?

Management is mainly symptomatic. In patients who are still currently on treatment, the causal agent should be stopped. See Figure 25.2 for suggested treatment algorithm.

Oxygen therapy precipitates bleomycin lung toxicity and exacerbates it when it occurs. Hence, careful assessment of oxygen levels with arterial blood gases is key. If hypoxic (<88%), controlled oxygen with a venturi mask should be used, aiming for oxygen saturation in the range of 88–92% SpO_2.[2] In type 1 respiratory failure in patients with malignancy who have undergone chemotherapy, there is some evidence to suggest that early non-invasive ventilation is associated with a better outcome.[8] We would therefore recommend early referral to the respiratory team to facilitate access to ventilatory support.

The management plan for steroids in suspected chemotherapy-induced lung toxicity is mainly based on observation.[9] However, it is reinforced by histological evidence of response in biopsy specimens.

In most cases the offending medication is stopped permanently, unless there is a strong reason otherwise.

Table 25.3 Common Toxicity Criteria to grade pneumonitis	
Grade 0	None
Grade 1	Radiographic changes but asymptomatic or symptoms not requiring steroids
Grade 2	Radiographic changes and requiring steroids or diuretics
Grade 3	Radiographic changes and requiring oxygen
Grade 4	Radiographic changes and requiring assisted ventilation

Figure 25.2 The following flow diagram is based on bleomycin as this is where the most evidence lies, but it can be used as a guide for most chemotherapy-induced lung damage.

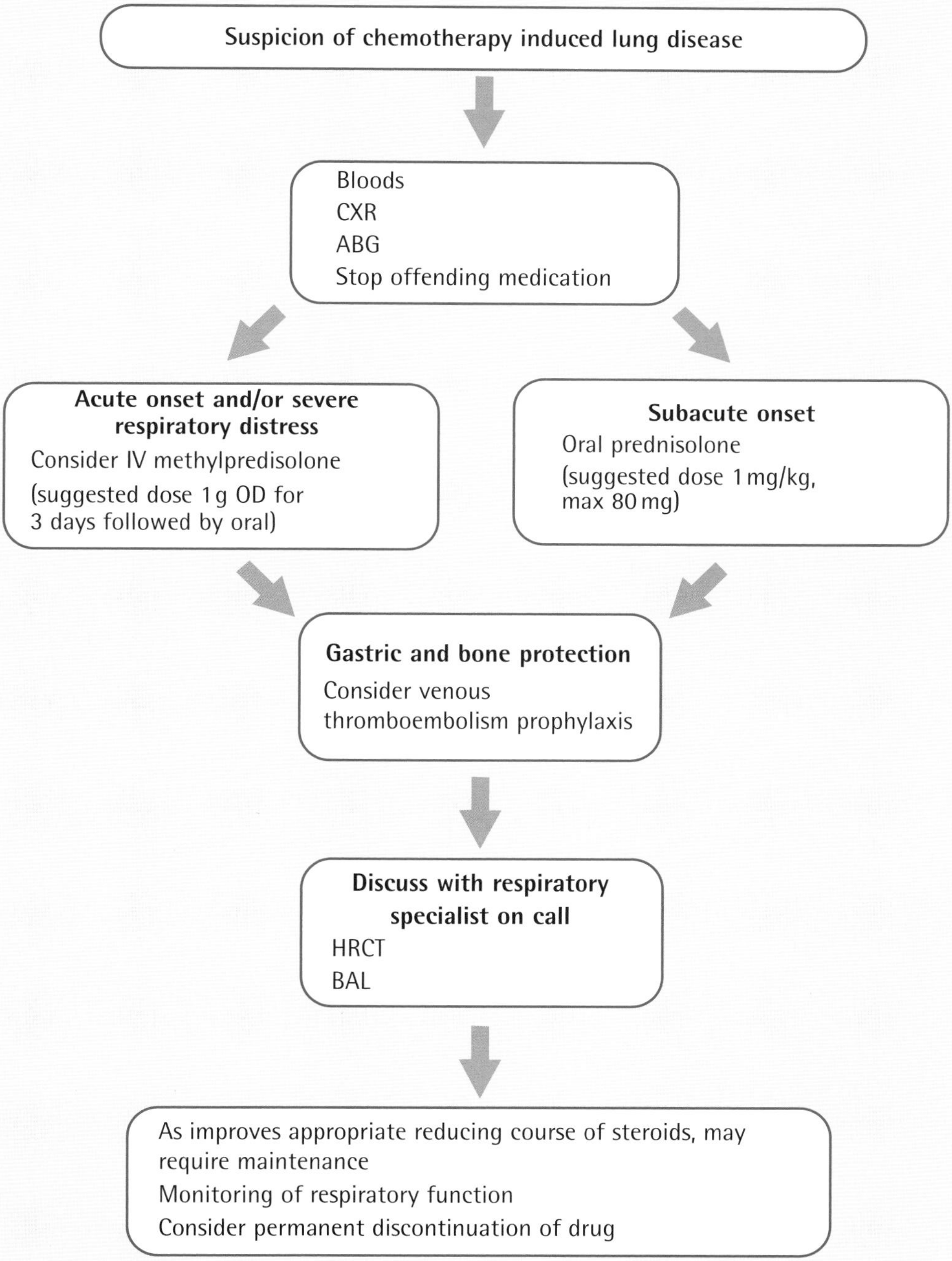

Suspicion of chemotherapy induced lung disease

Bloods
CXR
ABG
Stop offending medication

Acute onset and/or severe respiratory distress
Consider IV methylpredisolone
(suggested dose 1 g OD for 3 days followed by oral)

Subacute onset
Oral prednisolone
(suggested dose 1 mg/kg, max 80 mg)

Gastric and bone protection
Consider venous thromboembolism prophylaxis

Discuss with respiratory specialist on call
HRCT
BAL

As improves appropriate reducing course of steroids, may require maintenance
Monitoring of respiratory function
Consider permanent discontinuation of drug

ABG, arterial blood gas; BAL, bronchoalveolar lavage; CXR, chest X-ray; HRCT, high-resolution computed tomography

Further reading

1 Limper AH. Chemotherapy-induced lung disease. *Clin Chest Med* 2004; **25**(1): 53–64.

2 O'Driscoll BR, Howard LS, Davison AG; on behalf of British Thoracic Society Emergency Oxygen Guideline Development Group. Guideline for emergency oxygen use in adult patients. *Thorax* 2008; **63**(Suppl VI): vi1–vi68. doi:10.1136/thx.2008.102947

3 Perry MC, editor. *The Chemotherapy Source Book.* 4th ed. Philadelphia: Lippincott Williams & Wilkins; 2008. (Updated 5th edition provides excellent additional reading.)

4 Vahid B, Marik PE. Pulmonary complications of novel antineoplastic agents for solid tumors. *Chest* 2008; **133**: 528–38.

5 O'Sullivan JM, Huddart RA, Norman AR, Nicholls J, Dearnaley DP, Horwich A. Predicting the risk of bleomycin lung toxicity in patients with germ-cell tumours. *Ann Oncol* 2003; **14**: 91–6.

6 White DA, Stover DE. Severe bleomycin-induced pneumonitis. Clinical features and response to corticosteroids. *Chest* 1984; **86**: 723–8.

7 Camus P, Bonniaud P, Fanton A, Camus C, Baudaun N, Foucher P. Drug-induced and iatrogenic infiltrative lung disease. *Clin Chest Med* 2004; **25**: 479–519.

8 Gristina GR, Antonelli M, Conti G, et al. Noninvasive versus invasive ventilation for acute respiratory failure in patients with hematologic malignancies: a 5-year multicenter observational survey. *Crit Care Med* 2011; **39**(10): 2232–9.

9 Maldonado F, Limper AH, Jett JR. Pulmonary toxicity associated with antineoplastic therapy: Molecularly targeted agents [Internet]. Waltham, Mass.: UpToDate; c.2011–13. [Last updated 27 Feb 2013]. Available from: www.uptodate.com/pulmonary-toxicity-associated-with-antineoplastic-therapy-molecularly-targeted-agents.

Complications of Radiotherapy

PROBLEM

26 Radiation Pneumonitis

Ahmed Hashmi, Isabel Syndikus

Case history

A 65-year-old woman with T2a N2 M0 squamous cell lung cancer of the left upper
lobe presents to the emergency department. She has a two-week history of
progressively worsening shortness of breath on exertion, and a dry cough. She
completed four weeks of radical radiotherapy two months ago.

What is radiation pneumonitis?

What are the risk factors for the formation of radiation pneumonitis?

How should a patient with radiation pneumonitis be managed?

Background

What is radiation pneumonitis?
Radiation-related lung toxicity is divided into early and late phases. Early-phase toxicity
is defined as radiation pneumonitis. Late-phase toxicity is defined as radiation-related
pulmonary fibrosis.

   Radiation pneumonitis usually develops two to three months after the completion of
radiotherapy, but it can on occasions develop within the first month after radiotherapy,

or up to six months after radiotherapy.[1] From 5% to 15% of patients who receive external beam radiotherapy for lung cancer will develop symptomatic radiation pneumonitis, and up to 10% of patients receiving adjuvant radiotherapy for breast cancer will be symptomatic. A larger percentage of patients will have radiological features of pneumonitis but will be asymptomatic.[1]

Ionizing radiation leads to direct cellular damage to normal lung tissue; it also causes upregulation of cytokines that mediate the inflammatory process that leads to pneumonitis.

Radiotherapy can damage epithelial and endothelial cells, which causes narrowing of the pulmonary vasculature and small vessel thrombosis. An inflammatory exudate is formed that leads to alveolar cell hyperplasia.

Shortness of breath is the commonest symptom present, and the severity can vary. Cough is less common and is usually non-productive. Occasionally there can also be low-grade fever.[2] In rare cases there are fine crackles and friction rubs on auscultation. However, quite often there are no clinical signs.

Radiation pneumonitis does not necessarily have to show any radiological features on chest X-ray. If any are present there can be localized interstitial shadowing visible, normally corresponding to the treatment field. Computed tomography (CT) scans of thorax will typically show ground glass attenuation within the area of irradiation. A symptom severity scoring system is shown in Table 26.1

Table 26.1	Radiation Therapy Oncology Group (RTOG) grading of radiation lung toxicity based on symptoms
Grade 1	Mild cough or mild shortness of breath on exertion; no clinical intervention required
Grade 2	Cough requiring narcotic-based antitussive (codeine linctus)
Grade 3	Severe cough not responsive to narcotic or shortness of breath at rest; requires ambulatory oxygen or corticosteroids
Grade 4	Continuous oxygen or assisted ventilation required
Grade 5	Fatal

What are the risk factors for the development of radiation pneumonitis?

There are a variety of factors associated with the increased risk of developing radiation pneumonitis.

Radiotherapy-related factors

The volume of lung irradiated is an important factor in the development of radiation pneumonitis. Thus the greater the volume of lung irradiated the greater the likelihood of developing lung damage.[3]

The mean dose to the normal lung can be a predictor in the development of radiation pneumonitis. The V20 is defined as the volume of normal lung minus the planned treated volume that receives more than 20 Gy. The percentage of lung receiving this volume is an important predictor for the development of radiation pneumonitis.[4]

Chemotherapy

Concomitant chemotherapy using agents with known pulmonary toxicities may exacerbate radiation-related lung injury. A higher rate of pulmonary toxicity has been noted with the combined use of agents such as mitomycin, bleomycin and taxanes. Unsurprisingly, concurrent chemotherapy is associated with an increased risk of radiation pneumonitis compared to the use of sequential chemotherapy.

Other risk factors

Poor performance status, reduced lung function and previous radiotherapy to the chest are all risk factors for the development of radiation pneumonitis.[5]

Use of tamoxifen concurrently with adjuvant radiotherapy for breast cancer is associated with an increased risk in the development of pulmonary fibrosis, though this risk is reduced if it is used sequentially.[6]

How should a patient with radiation pneumonitis be managed?

Any patient presenting with respiratory symptoms, e.g. shortness of breath, should be thoroughly assessed. It is important to rule out other causes, such as pneumonia, pulmonary embolus, progression of disease and symptomatic anaemia. Radiation pneumonitis should only be diagnosed if other possible causes of these symptoms are first excluded, and the symptoms develop within an adequate timeframe when radiation pneumonitis is known to develop.

Corticosteroids have been the mainstay of management for radiation pneumonitis. Studies in mice have shown that the administration of corticosteroids during irradiation reduces the risk of abnormality in lung function.[7] Corticosteroids are thought to lessen the extent of radiation pneumonitis by reducing inflammation; this is done by the inhibition of tumour necrosis factor-induced cell damage. To begin with, 60 mg of prednisolone should be given with adequate gastric protection using a proton pump inhibitor (PPI) cover for at least two weeks. The dose is then gradually reduced over a period of 12 weeks.

Supportive care with oxygen may be required, and if fibrosis develops then long-term oxygenation might be necessary.

Conclusion

The patient presenting with shortness of breath following radiotherapy should be assessed for common causes of these symptoms. Radiation pneumonitis should mainly be a diagnosis of exclusion. Supportive care along with the use of corticosteroids is the mainstay of management.

Further reading

1   McDonald S, Rubin P, Phillips TL. Injury to the lung from cancer therapy: clinical syndromes, measurable endpoints, and potential scoring system. *Int J Radiat Oncol Biol Phys* 1995; **31**: 1187–203.

2   Abratt RP, Morgan GW, Gilvestri G, Willcox P. Pumonary complications of radiation therapy. *Clin Chest Med* 2004; **25**: 167–77.

3   Morgan GW, Breit SN. Radiation and the lung: revaluation of the mechanisms mediating pulmonary injury. *Int J Radiat Oncol Biol Phys* 1995; **31**: 361–9.

4   Fay M, Tan A, Fisher R, MacManus M, Wirth A, Ball D. Dose-volume histogram analysis as predictor of radiation pneumonitis in primary lung cancer patients treated with radiotherapy. *Int J Radiat Oncol Biol Phys* 2005; **61**: 1355–63.

5   Robnett TJ, Machtay M, Vines EF, McKenna MG, Algazy KM, McKenna WG. Factors predicting severe radiation pneumonitis in patients receiving definitive chemoradiation for lung cancer. *Int J Radiat Oncol Biol Phys* 2000; **48**: 89–94.

6   Varga Z, Cserháti A, Kelemen G, Boda K, ThurzóL, Kahán Z. Role of systemic therapy in the development of lung sequelae after conformal radiotherapy in breast cancer patients. *Int J Radiat Oncol Biol Phys* 2011; 80: 1109–16.

7   Gross NJ, Narine KR, Wade R. Protective effect of corticosteroids on radiation pneumonitis in mice. *Radiat Res* 1988; **113**: 112–9.

27 Radiation-Induced Head and Neck Mucositis

Mary Anthonypillai, Isabel Syndikus

Case history

A patient with a T3 N2a M0 hypopharyngeal cancer is admitted to the emergency department on a Saturday. The patient is three weeks into his six-week chemoradiation treatment. He has found it difficult to swallow due to pain for a number of days, and he is unable to swallow solids or liquids. On examination of his oral cavity his mucous membranes are inflamed and there are several ulcers present.

Why does radiation-induced mucositis occur?

How should patients with oral mucositis be assessed?

How should patients with radiation-induced oral mucositis be managed?

Background

Mucositis refers to the inflammation and/or ulcerative lesions of the oral and or gastrointestinal (GI) tract.[1] It can occur as a side effect of both radiotherapy and chemotherapy treatment. Mucositis occurs when radiotherapy is directed at or near to the oral cavity or GI tract.

Radiotherapy is an important component of the management of head and neck cancers, hence oral mucositis is a common and expected side effect of radiotherapy to this region. Over 80% of patients receiving radical doses of radiotherapy to the head and neck region suffer with severe oral mucositis.[1] Patients can experience oral ulcers and varying degrees of odynophagia.

Typically, patients do not experience any symptoms in the first week of a 4–7-week treatment schedule, and mucositis is often delayed, becoming more severe towards the latter part of treatment. It is important to warn patients that their symptoms will not clear on completion of treatment and that it may take several weeks for the symptoms of mucositis to resolve.

Why does radiation-induced mucositis occur?

Although a high proportion of patients treated radically for head and neck cancers develop mucositis, severity varies from patient to patient. This suggests a genetic component, although further research is needed to establish the key factors.

The pathogenesis of mucositis is also an ongoing area of research. The basic stages thought to be involved in the pathogenesis of both oral and GI mucositis are similar and are outlined in Figure 27.1.

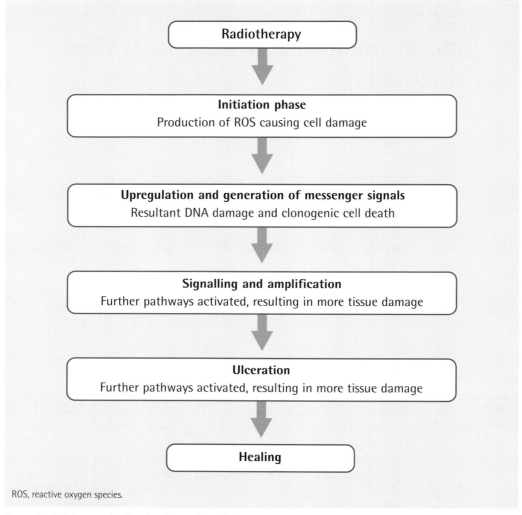

Figure 27.1 Pathogenesis of oral and gastrointestinal mucositis. Adapted from ref. 2.

How should patients with mucositis be assessed?

Mucositis is an expected side effect of radical head and neck radiotherapy; consequently, patients should be assessed prior to, during and after treatment.

Patients should be assessed by a dentist prior to starting treatment to optimize education concerning oral hygiene, and to complete any necessary dental work before starting treatment. Oral hygiene is particularly important for those patients undergoing chemoradiation to help prevent infection.

Patients who are unable to manage oral nutrition may require dietary supplements and/or a percutaneous endoscopic gastrostomy (PEG) or a nasogastric (NG) tube to meet their nutritional needs. For this reason, all patients should be assessed by a dietician.

Two grading systems for mucositis are used in clinical practice: these are the World Health Organization (WHO) scale for oral mucositis and the National Cancer Institute (NCI) Common Terminology Criteria for Adverse Events (CTCAE) scales. These are illustrated in Table 27.1.

Table 27.1 Two grading systems for mucositis used in clinical practice

Grade	WHO scale	CTCAE scale
0	No oral mucositis	–
1	Erythema and soreness	Asymptomatic or mild symptoms; no intervention required
2	Ulcers, able to eat solids	Moderate pain not interfering with oral intake; modified diet required
3	Ulcers, requires liquid diet	Severe pain interfering with oral intake
4	Ulcers, alimentation not possible	Life-threatening consequences, urgent intervention required
5	–	Death

CTCAE, Common Terminology Criteria for Adverse Events; WHO, World Health Organization.

How should patients with radiation-induced oral mucositis be managed?

Management of oral mucositis is largely supportive and should entail a multidisciplinary approach with early involvement of specialist nurses, dentists and dieticians. The basic principles of management are:

1. **Patient education** – Advice on oral hygiene should be given. If significant mucositis is expected, patients should be seen by a dentist to advise on how to maintain good oral hygiene. There is limited evidence as to what constitutes good oral hygiene. Systematic protocol-driven regimes involving the use of a soft toothbrush, bland rinses and moisturizers are considered good practice.[3]

2. **Dietary support** – The patient should be weighed and assessed with regard to their nutritional needs on a regular basis. Patients may require NG or PEG feeding.

3. **Analgesia** – Regular analgesia, that may include opiates, should be provided early and often. This helps to maintain an oral diet for as long as possible.

It is important to emphasize that chemoradiation should continue despite severe symptoms of mucositis. If the patient presents at the emergency department, the treating oncology team should be contacted as soon as possible so that arrangements can be made to continue with treatment.

Although the basic principles of management of radiation-induced oral mucositis are widely agreed upon, many of the medications prescribed often have little evidence to support their use. As a result, clinical practice guidelines have been established to assess the efficacy of mucositis management and make recommendations based on the available evidence (Table 27.2).[3–5]

Table 27.2 Clinical practice guidelines for oral mucositis management

Oral hygiene is considered good clinical practice, despite little evidence that it aids in mucositis management.

Benzydamine hydrochloride oral rinse – reduces frequency, severity and pain of oral mucositis.

The use of oral sucralfate, chlorhexidine mouthwashes and antibacterial mouthwashes is not recommended.

There is insufficient evidence to recommend the use of amifostine in the treatment of oral mucositis.

Computed tomography (CT) conformal radiotherapy or intensity-modulated radiotherapy are considered good practice.

Conclusion

Mucositis is an expected side effect of radiotherapy. The treatment of mucositis should involve early and continued support by the multidisciplinary team. The oncology team treating the patient should be contacted at the earliest time to ensure optimal management and communication, and to ensure that treatment can continue wherever possible.

Further reading

1   Peterson DE, Bensadon R-J, Roila F. Management of oral and gastrointestinal mucositis: ESMO clinical practice guidelines. *Ann Oncol* 2011; **22**(6 suppl): vi78–vi84.

2   Sonis ST, Elting LS, Keefe D, *et al.* Perspectives on cancer therapy-induced mucosal injury. Pathogenesis, measurement, epidemiology and consequences for patients. *Cancer* 2004; **100**: 1995–2011.

3   Rubenstein EB, Peterson DE, Schubert M, *et al.* Clinical practice guidelines for the prevention of cancer therapy-induced oral and gastrointestinal mucositis. *Cancer* 2004; **100**(9 suppl): 2026–46.

4   Keefe DM, Schubert MM, Elting LS *et al.* Update. Clinical practice guidelines for the prevention and treatment of mucositis. *Cancer* 2007; **109**: 820–31.

5   Hensley ML, Hagerty KL, Kewalramani T, *et al.* American Society of Clinical Oncology practice guideline update: use of chemotherapy and radiation therapy protectants. *J Clin Oncol* 2009; **27**: 127–45.

28 Management of Radiotherapy–Related Acute Skin Toxicity in the Acute Oncology Setting

Anthony Pope, Isabel Syndikus

Case history

A 54-year-old woman who completed a fractionated course of radiotherapy to her breast seven days ago presents with redness and tenderness/pain in the breast accompanied by general malaise.

What is radiotherapy-related acute skin toxicity?

How should the patient be assessed?

What else should be excluded?

How can you manage the problem?

Background

What is radiotherapy-related acute skin toxicity?

The cells in the basal layer of the epidermis constantly divide to form the upper layers of the skin, with a turnover time of about 25 days. Radiation damages the DNA of stem cells in the basal layer, resulting in apoptosis, mitotic cell death and an inflammatory response. The sequential nature of a course of radiotherapy interrupts ongoing repair processes, thus consolidating injury.[1,2]

Acute skin toxicity secondary to radiotherapy usually occurs at 12–14 days and the severity is dependent upon the following:

- Patient-related factors:
  - treatment site (head and neck cancer, breast cancer, vulval cancer, anal canal cancer and skin cancer)
  - radiation sensitivity (related to genetic predisposition)
  - comorbidity (pre-existing skin infiltration by cancer, chronic oedema, ulceration or infection)
  - obesity (skin folds are more at risk).
- Treatment-related factors:
  - radiation dose (high-dose treatments cause more problems)
  - radiotherapy beam energy (kilovoltage photons or electrons)
  - use of bolus (increases dose to skin)
  - immobilization masks
  - concurrent chemotherapy.

Symptoms of skin toxicity include: itching, discomfort or pain, erythema, ulceration, scab formation and functional impairment.

The majority of data on radiotherapy-induced acute skin toxicity comes from patients receiving radiotherapy to the breast region and head and neck region. Acute skin toxicity can also be a serious problem in anal/lower rectal and some gynaecological treatments (dose is concentrated in folds), and is an expected problem in skin cancer treatments. Owing to the likely distribution of radiation beams and subsequent dosage, severe acute skin toxicities are rare in other tumour groups.

In most patients who have 4–6 weeks of radiotherapy, skin side effects will develop during the course. In shorter courses of therapy the acute toxicity can occur after completion of the course, and this can cause alarm.

How should the patient be assessed?

Skin changes look like sunburn or burns, and they occur only in the treated area, often with a very sharp demarcation from normal skin. A number of grading systems exist to help assess the severity of an acute skin toxicity and give guidance for management. Commonly used in the UK are the Radiation Therapy Oncology Group (RTOG) Acute Radiation Morbidity Scoring Criteria (Table 28.1).[3,4] Desquamation refers to the loss of the epithelium exposing the underlying dermal layer.

Table 28.1 Radiation Therapy Oncology Group (RTOG) Acute Radiation Morbidity Scoring Criteria

RTOG grade	Description	Symptoms
1	Follicular, faint or dull erythema/epilation/ dry desquamation	Decreased sweating, feeling of heat
2	Tender or bright erythema, patchy moist desquamation/moderate oedema	Pruritus, burning sensation, tenderness, tightness
3	Confluent, moist desquamation other than skin folds, pitting oedema	Severe pain, increased risk of infection, impaired mobility
4	Ulceration, haemorrhage, necrosis	As above

Grade 3 or 4 acute toxicity, as in this case study description, can occur after completion of treatment. In this setting the responsible clinical oncologist may not be aware of the problem; it may be helpful to contact the treating team or acute oncology team for advice.

Assessment of patients

- Examination of the skin

- Check for underlying seroma

- If there is a moist exudate then swab for microscopy, culture and sensitivity

- Full blood count, including differential

- Blood cultures if systemically unwell or neutropenic.

What else should be excluded?

Often patients with severe acute skin toxicity also have concurrent mucositis and other symptoms such as cystitis or diarrhoea. The management of the skin is part of an overall strategy. The loss of the skin as a barrier predisposes to infection; in extensive cases, skin loss can increase fluid loss, contributing to electrolyte imbalances, and affect temperature regulation.

Differentiation from cellulitis

Secondary infections (cellulitis) are common in ulcerated wounds. It is important to note that patients on chemotherapy, or who have recently completed chemotherapy and have a low neutrophil count, might not express signs despite infection. In addition, patients with skin breakdown and exudate in the groins, axillae and inframammary folds are prone to fungal infections and this differential diagnosis must be considered.

Secondary infections should be suspected if the following signs or symptoms are observed:

- purulent discharge
- prior infections after surgery
- erythema in the first 10 days of treatment
- significant pain and oedema
- other symptoms of infection; malaise, fever, raised white blood cell count

How can you manage the problem?

Systematic reviews and surveys of UK practice in the management of acute skin toxicity have demonstrated a wide variation across different oncology centres. There is little evidence of effectiveness, and the trials represent small cohort studies only. In addition, those that have demonstrated statistically significant benefits have rarely been validated

Table 28.2 General principles of radiotherapy-induced acute skin toxicity

Use a simple moisturizer such as aqueous cream for the intact skin in the treatment area. Radiation inhibits sebaceous and sweat gland function.

Avoid additional skin irritation: perfumed cosmetic products, excessive washing, scratching and rubbing, sun exposure.

Continue gentle washing of area with water; use a medicated wash, aqueous cream or mild soap as tolerated.

Use loose-fitting clothing and a soft breast prosthesis if appropriate.

Malnourished patients benefit from nutritional support, which improves skin healing.

Use a weak topical steroid, such as 1% hydrocortisone cream, on unbroken skin and dry desquamation.

In moist desquamation, avoid creams; use dry non-absorbent, hydrogel or hydrocolloid dressings if there is little wound exudate. For heavily exudating wounds use absorbent foam dressings. Involve a tissue viability nurse if appropriate.

Provide appropriate analgesia via the WHO analgesic ladder.

A topical gel combined with analgesic agents such as diamorphine have been used to good effect for painful ulcers.

Treat bacterial and fungal infection with oral or intravenous antibiotics or antifungal drugs according to sensitivity. In the absence of symptoms, normal skin flora bacteria require no treatment.

by repeat studies and therefore are not widely accepted in practice.[4-6] Principles of management are similar to those for the management of burns (Table 28.2) and the acute oncology team can facilitate discussion with the site-specific multidisciplinary team.

Impediments to skin healing

Radiotherapy-related skin toxicity normally heals within 4–6 weeks after completion of the treatment. Severe acute toxicity and ulceration may take longer. A combination of internal and external factors can delay healing of the skin:

- Comorbidities: peripheral vascular disease, diabetes, arteriosclerosis
- Increasing age: reduced metabolic rate, poorer circulation and nutritional deficits, structural changes
- Advanced malignancy: cachexia, malnutrition, altered angiogenesis
- Medication: steroids suppress fibroblast function and would healing; cytotoxics affect re-epithelialization, immune suppression
- Wound desiccation: dry wounds heal slower than those in a moist environment
- Maceration: excess exudate can cause the softening of the surrounding skin and breakdown leading to wound enlargement
- Infection: bacteria release enzymes into the skin, causing breakdown; they compete with the healing cells for nutrients
- Site: areas with poor blood supply such as the distal end of limbs are prone to delayed or incomplete healing

Conclusion

The majority of patients undergoing radical radiotherapy will have acute skin toxicity. Good skin care can reduce the severity of acute toxicity and facilitate healing, thus improving patients' quality of life and psychological wellbeing. Modern radiotherapy techniques such as intensity-modulated radiation therapy (IMRT) can reduce the problem. Conversely, the increasing use of concurrent chemoradiotherapy, and the use of shorter fraction number combined with larger fraction size, may exacerbate acute skin toxicity.

Further reading

1   Hymes SR, Strom EA, Fife C. Radiation dermatitis: clinical presentation, pathophysiology, and treatment. *J Am Acad Dermatol* 2006; **54**: 28–46.

2   Denham JW, Hauer-Jensen M. The radiotherapeutic injury – a complex 'wound'. *Radiother Oncol* 2002; **63**: 129–45.

3   Cox JD, Stetz J, Pajak TF. Toxicity criteria of the Radiation Therapy Oncology Group (RTOG) and the European Organization for Research and Treatment of Cancer (EORTC). *Int J Radiat Oncol Biol Phys* 1995; **31**(5): 1341–6.

4   Harris R, Probst H, Beardmore C, et al. Radiotherapy skin care: a survey of practice in the UK. *Radiography* 2012; **18**(1): 21–7.

5   Kumar S, Juresic E, Barton M, Shafiq J. Management of skin toxicity during radiation therapy: a review of the evidence. *J Med Imag Radiat Oncol* 2010; **54**: 264–79.

6   Salvo N, Barnes E, van Draanen J, *et al.* Prophylaxis and management of acute radiation-induced skin reactions: systematic review of the literature. *Curr Oncol* 2010; **17**(4): 94–112.

29 Toxicity Related to Pelvic Radiotherapy

Mary Anthonypillai, Isabel Syndikus

Case history

A 60-year-old man is admitted with diarrhoea. He has T3 N1 M0 rectal carcinoma and is receiving long-course chemoradiotherapy. Prior to the start of treatment the patient opened his bowels twice daily. The patient is now two weeks into his treatment and is opening his bowels six times daily. He is severely fatigued.

What are the acute side effects of pelvic radiotherapy?

How would you manage a patient with acute side effects from pelvic radiotherapy?

What are the late side effects of pelvic radiotherapy?

Background

Pelvic radiotherapy is used in the treatment of many cancers including rectal carcinoma, prostate cancer and cervical tumours. Directing radiation at the pelvis results in a number of different side effects, which largely relate to normal tissue damage. Advances in radiotherapy have resulted in less normal tissue damage and, as a result, fewer treatment-related side-effects.[1]

What are the acute side effects of pelvic radiotherapy?

Bowel toxicity

Bowel frequency and consistency can be affected by radiotherapy. Patients can also pass mucus or blood during treatment and often experience tenesmus.

Intestinal permeability alters during radiotherapy as a result of gastrointestinal mucositis. The pathogenesis is thought to be the same as that of oral mucositis (see section on mucositis). Certain factors are known to increase the likelihood of bowel toxicity and should be noted prior to commencing treatment (Table 29.1).

Table 29.1 Risk factors for bowel toxicity after radiation therapy for prostate cancer. (Adapted from ref. 1.)	
Advanced age	History of prior abdominal surgery
Large rectal volume	Pre-existing diabetes mellitus
Haemorrhoids	
Inflammatory bowel disease	

Bladder toxicity

Patients may experience 'cystitis-like' symptoms such as dysuria, increased frequency and urinary urgency. Male patients undergoing pelvic radiotherapy for prostate cancer frequently notice a reduced urinary flow.

Skin toxicity

The likelihood of skin toxicity depends upon the site of the radiotherapy target volume. Skin toxicity is uncommon in the treatment of prostate cancer and high rectal tumours. However, it can be severe in the treatment of low rectal, vulval tumours and tumours involving the anal margin.

How would you manage a patient with side effects from pelvic radiotherapy?

A change in bowel habit is an expected side-effect, but if any doubt exists as to the cause of diarrhoea then stool samples should be sent for culture and sensitivities. If there has been recent antibiotic treatment it is advisable to check for *Clostridium difficile* infection.

Management of acute bowel toxicity is supportive and comprises adequate hydration and antidiarhoeal agents such as loperamide and codeine phosphate. Regular blood parameters should be checked to ensure electrolytes are replaced, neutropenia is monitored and red cell transfusion is not required. Tenesmus can sometimes be helped by a short course of steroid enemas.

Patients with urinary symptoms may avoid drinking in an attempt to reduce their urinary frequency. It is important to encourage oral hydration with liquids. Sensible measures the patient can take themselves are avoidance of diuretics such as tea and alcohol; not drinking in the few hours before sleep can help if nocturia is a problem. Male patients with urinary outflow symptoms may benefit from by alpha-blockers such as tamsulosin.

Management of skin toxicity is covered in a separate case study (*see* Chapter 28).

What are the late side effects of pelvic radiotherapy?

Sexual function and fertility

Female patients receiving a significant dose of radiotherapy to the pelvis will be warned about vaginal stenosis. Vaginal dilators of various sizes are provided for the patient to use after their radiotherapy has completed. Vaginal dryness can also occur.

Female patients receiving pelvic radiotherapy often become infertile as a result of treatment. This should be discussed with the patient prior to the start of treatment.

Male patients receiving treatment for prostate cancer may become impotent. It is difficult to know how many men are affected by radiotherapy, as many have had hormonal treatment or have other comorbidities that can also cause impotence. Patients should be referred to their general practitioner or an appropriate specialist for management.

Bowel toxicity

Patients may notice a permanent change in bowel habit following radiotherapy. Symptoms tend to occur in the first two years following treatment and include frequency and urgency.[2] Occasionally, patients experience rectal bleeding. Patients with persistent rectal bleeding should always be investigated for a possible second malignancy.

Bladder toxicity

Patients may experience a change to their normal frequency and flow. Long-term urinary incontinence and severe urinary symptoms are rare.[2–4]

Conclusion

Radiotherapy to the pelvis can cause a number of different side effects related to the effects of radiation on normal tissue. Many of the side effects result in both physical and psychological distress, and patients should have continued assessment and support during and after treatment.

Further reading

1   Budäus L, Bolla M, Bossi A *et al.* Functional outcomes and complications following radiation therapy for prostate cancer: a critical analysis of the literature. *Eur Urol* 2012; **61**(1): 112–27.

2   Phan J, Swanson DA, Levy LB, Kudchadker RJ, Bruno TL, Frank SJ. Late rectal complications after prostate brachytherapy for localized prostate cancer: incidence and management. *Cancer* 2009; **115**: 1827–39.

3   Zietman AL, DeSilvio ML, Slater JD, *et al.* Comparison of conventional-dose vs high-dose conformal radiation therapy in clinically localized adenocarcinoma of the prostate: a randomized controlled trial. *JAMA* 2005; **294**: 1233–9.

4   Williams SG, Zietman AL. Does radical treatment have a role in the management of low-risk prostate cancer? The place for brachytherapy and external beam radiotherapy. *World J Urol* 2008; **26**: 447–56.

5   Williams SG, Millar JL, Duchesne GM, Dally MJ, Royce PL, Snow RM. Factors predicting for urinary morbidity following [125]iodine transperineal prostate brachytherapy. *Radiother Oncol* 2004; **73**: 33–8.

6   Hanna L, Crosby T, Macbeth F, editors. *Practical Clinical Oncology.* Cambridge University Press; Mar 2008. 512p.

30 Central Nervous System Toxicity of Radiotherapy

Anthony Pope

Case history

A 45-year-old man has recently completed chemoradiation for a glioblastoma multiforme and is taking adjuvant temozolomide. The patient presents following a seizure at home and has residual right-sided lower limb weakness. He is complaining of a frontal headache and nausea.

What causes CNS toxicity after radiotherapy?

What is the differential diagnosis?

What are the common side effects encountered following CNS radiotherapy?

How should post-radiotherapy complications be managed?

Background

What causes CNS toxicity after radiotherapy?

Central nervous system (CNS) toxicity of radiotherapy is divided into three phases of damage: acute, consequential and late. The majority of problems likely to be encountered in the acute oncology setting are acute and consequential (continuing after completion of radiation); late is classed as over 90 days after completion of treatment.

Acute toxicity is thought to be secondary to blood–brain barrier disruption, glial cell damage and swelling. Radiation damages DNA and hence cellular structure, both directly and also indirectly via the production of free radicals. Glial cells, such as oligodendrocytes, experience higher rates of cell turnover and are therefore subject to damage by fractionated courses of treatment. Radiation does not significantly damage the neurons themselves. Subsequent demyelination, altered cytokine production and apoptosis can lead to loss of function. Chemotherapy prior to radiotherapy can increase neurotoxicity.

Longer-term complications are a combination of the above effects along with radiotherapy damage to the vascular structures of the CNS that manifest as dysregulated cell division.[1] This results primarily in a reduction in cognitive ability and the onset of dementia-type symptoms.

What is the differential diagnosis?

Prognosis for CNS malignancy is highly variable and may range from 6 to15 months in high-grade glioblastoma, whereas median survival in metastatic CNS disease is only four months.[2,3] A significant proportion of patients may also undergo CNS radiotherapy in a setting with a more favourable prognosis, including low-grade primary CNS tumours and prophylactic therapy in small-cell lung cancer.

Neurological deterioration can result from radiotherapy toxicity or disease progression. The differential diagnosis, investigation and management of individual patients is directed by the underlying diagnosis, treatment timing and intent. Direct contact with the acute oncology team and treating neuro-oncologist will often represent the most important aspect of patient care.

In the setting of primary brain tumours there is a cohort of patients who present during or shortly after treatment with side effects directly attributable to radiotherapy. However, caution must be observed because this group have often recently undergone surgery. Therefore, they are prone to complications secondary to structural disturbance, such as bleeding, infarcts, and raised intracranial pressure due to cerebrospinal fluid (CSF) obstruction. In addition, the cancer itself predisposes to these complications. Particular care must be taken with those patients on long-term steroids, as these will mask signs of infection by suppressing fever and pus production. In the setting of a cranial flap and connected surgical cavity, undetected infections can prove rapidly fatal. Consequently, a low threshold for imaging should be applied, and a neurological opinion sought.

The treatment pathway illustrated in Figure 30.1 can be adapted for both metastatic and adjuvant patients, as the primary concern is to rule out complications that can be addressed by surgical management. In the metastatic setting, performance status and extent of systemic disease should heavily influence the extent of investigation; however, radiation doses are lower and so major toxicities are less common.

Radiation Therapy Oncology Group grading
Toxicity can be defined using the Radiation Therapy Oncology Group (RTOG) grading, and this can facilitate communication and management (Table 30.1).

Table 30.1 Radiation Therapy Oncology Group (RTOG) toxicity grading

Grade 1	Fully functional status (i.e. able to work) with minor neurological findings, no medication needed
Grade 2	Neurological findings present sufficient to require home care; nursing assistance may be required; medications including steroids/antiseizure agents may be required
Grade 3	Neurological findings requiring hospitalization for initial management
Grade 4	Paralysis, coma, frequent seizures despite medication

What are the common side effects of CNS radiotherapy and how should they be managed?

Encephalopathy
In rare cases, when large areas of the brain are treated, symptoms of encephalopathy can manifest themselves. This is typically characterized by headache, drowsiness, often a return of prior symptoms, increased seizure frequency, or new seizures. This is thought to be due to disruption of the blood–brain barrier leading to increased cerebral oedema and

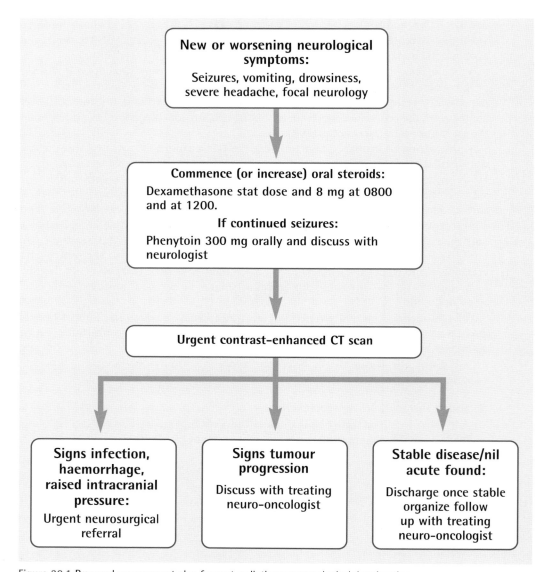

Figure 30.1 Proposed management plan for post-radiotherapy neurological deterioration.

subsequent raised intracranial pressure. With modern radiotherapy fractionation and dosage the frequency of encephalopathy is typically 5% of those treated.[4] Encephalopathic features typically occur within the first two weeks of treatment. In those patients with primary brain tumours, debulking surgery often leaves a flap within the skull vault which can mitigate the symptoms by allowing expansion and so reducing the pressure.

Management is with commencement (or increased dose) of corticosteroids, e.g. dexamethasone 8–16 mg daily. This will usually control seizures if they are a problem, but if unsuccessful then antiepileptic medication such as phenytoin is indicated.

Nausea/vomiting

Nausea is encountered in the acute setting, rarely of a severity to induce vomiting. This will usually respond to antiemetics, and low-dose steroids can be effective. If concurrent chemotherapy is administered then this will increase the likelihood of this complication.

Somnolence syndrome

Cranial irradiation can lead to excessive fatigue. This has been characterized by a syndrome which occurs 6 to 12 weeks after completion of radiotherapy. In most cases it is mild, with minimal effects on activity levels; however, in rare cases a more severe form may develop, possibly secondary to transient demyelination. This is usually self-limiting and resolves over a period of a several weeks. There is no proven intervention for this problem, although steroids may offer some benefit.[5]

Hair loss

Although not clinically concerning this has a considerable psychological impact on patients – all patients will have hair loss to some degree. In most patients undergoing whole-brain radiotherapy hair will return after a period of months. With partial brain treatment the extent of hair loss is often less, but, unfortunately, due to the higher dose used it is often permanent.

Skin reaction

A transient inflammation of the skin may occur but is usually mild and self-limiting.

Necrosis and pseudo-progression

Necrosis and pseudo-progression are two late effects of radiation that may give the imaging characteristics of progressive tumour when in fact none has occurred. This can occur in up to 20% of patients treated with concurrent temozolomide and radiotherapy for glioblastoma.[6] Therefore, caution should be employed when informing this cohort of their results without specialist neuro-oncology input. Management of symptomatic radiation necrosis involves steroids and observation, or surgery in extreme cases.

Long-term complications

The primary toxicity of concern in those who may survive long term, such as patients with CNS non-Hodgkin lymphoma and particularly the paediatric population, is that of cognitive decline. This is detectable with variable intensity in up to a third of long-term survivors.

Conclusion

The acute presentation of patients following CNS radiation treatment represents a complex treatment scenario that is often multifactorial and involves the primary tumour, radiotherapy, and patient factors. Stabilization through increased steroid dose, symptom control and brain imaging should be combined with early input from the acute oncology team and communication with the specialist neuro-oncology multidisciplinary team.

Further reading

1   Belka C, Budach W, Kortmann RD, Bamberg M. Radiation induced CNS toxicity – molecular and cellular mechanisms. *Br J Cancer* 2001; **85**(9): 1233–9.

2   Khuntia D, Brown P, Li J, Mehta MP. Whole-brain radiotherapy in the management of brain metastasis. *J Clin Oncol* 2006; **24**: 1295–304.

3   Stupp R, Mason WP, van den Bent MJ, *et al.* Radiotherapy plus concomitant and adjuvant temozolomide for glioblastoma. *N Engl J Med* 2005; **352**(10): 987–96.

4   Yaccov R, Allen L , Issam N. Radiation dose-volume effects in brain [QUANTEC organ-specific paper]. *Int J Radiat Oncol Biol Phys* 2010; **76**(3 Suppl): S20–S27.

5   Powell C, Guerrero D, Sardell S. Somnolence syndrome in patients receiving radical radiotherapy for primary brain tumours: a prospective study. *Radiother Oncol* 2011; **100**: 131–6.

6   Brandsma D, Stalpers L, Taal W, Simnia P, van den Bent MJ. Clinical features, mechanisms, and management of pseudoprogression in malignant gliomas. *Lancet Oncol* 2008; **9**(5): 453–61.

7   Radiation Therapy Oncology Group. *Acute radiation morbidity scoring criteria* [Internet]. Philadelphia: RTOG; c.2013. Available from: www.rtog.org/ResearchAssociates/ AdverseEventReporting/ AcuteRadiationMorbidityScoringCriteria.aspx

Complications of Cancer

PROBLEM

31 Spinal Cord Compression

Peter Robson, Martin Wilby

Case History

A 65-year-old man presents with thoracic back pain, tiredness and a 24-hour history of leg weakness (Medical Research Council Scale muscle power 4). His back pain has been present for three months. An urgent whole-spine MRI reveals a single-level lesion at T5 causing cord compression (Figure 31.1). There is no significant past medical history and examination reveals no other abnormality.

What underlying malignancies would you consider in your differential diagnosis?

What is the immediate management?

What are the options for treatment and how do you assess which is the most appropriate?

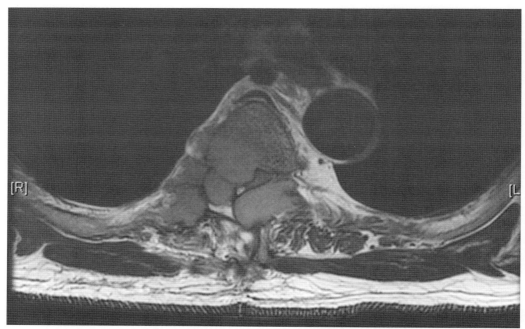

Figure 31.1 Axial T2-weighted (fluid white) magnetic resonance image showing soft tissue metastasis causing cord compression at the mid-thoracic level.

Background

What underlying malignancies would you consider in your differential diagnosis?

Prostate cancer is the most likely diagnosis in men of this age group. It frequently presents at diagnosis with signs and symptoms of metastatic disease, and may present with metastatic spinal cord compression (MSCC). The diagnosis of prostate cancer would usually be confirmed by clinical examination of the prostate and elevated PSA level. Other common primary sites would include lung cancer and myeloma, with renal and thyroid cancer being less common. In women, the breast would be the most common site of origin.

Although it would be uncommon for lymphoma to present in this way it must always be considered in the differential diagnosis. If lymphoma is suspected then a biopsy must be undertaken prior to commencement of any steroids. Treatment with corticosteroids prior to biopsy may prevent a diagnosis being made.

What is the immediate management?

Any patient presenting with signs or symptoms suggesting MSCC should be treated as outlined in the National Institute for Health and Care Excellence (NICE) guidance CG75 (see also Figure 31.2).[1] They should be laid flat to avoid further damage from a potentially unstable spine and to improve perfusion of the spinal cord. High-dose steroids are recommended (16 mg dexamethasone daily with proton pump inhibitor cover) to reduce oedema and inhibit prostaglandin synthesis. These should be used unless contraindicated, or if there is a high clinical suspicion of lymphoma. Clinical trials have shown no statistical benefit and increased side effects with very high-dose steroids (100 mg) and their use is therefore not recommended.[2] Appropriate analgesia should be given to the patient.

MSCC is an oncological emergency and should be diagnosed from an MRI scan of the whole spine done within 24 hours of neurological signs/symptoms developing.[1,3] Following diagnosis, rapid treatment is required as extrinsic compression of the spinal cord may lead to irreversible damage and permanent neurological deficit. Initial signs are due to vasogenic oedema of the cord, which may be reversible with steroids and laying the patient supine. If the oedema progresses to ischaemic death of neurons (either indirectly via vascular damage, or directly by compression) then any deficit will become permanent. Once a patient has lost all motor power for >48 hours there is unlikely to be any recovery of useful function.

Contact should be made with your regional MSCC coordinator immediately following diagnosis to allow rapid management decisions to be made and appropriate transfer for specialist treatment.[1]

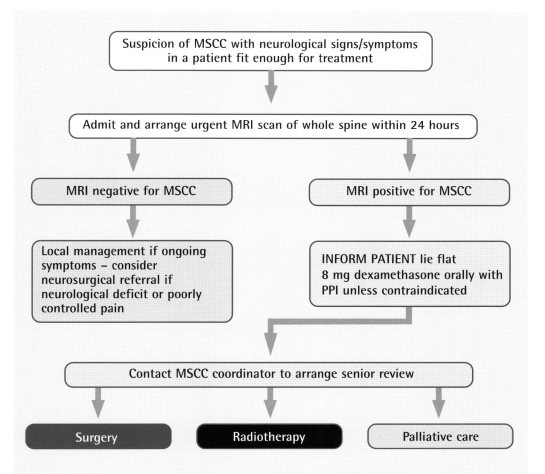

Figure 31.2 Flow chart for diagnosis and treatment of MSCC. PPI, proton pump inhibitor.

What are the treatment options and how do you assess which is the most appropriate?

The definitive treatment options for a patient presenting with MSCC are surgery or radiotherapy. However, careful consideration must first be given to whether the patient is deemed fit enough for transfer and treatment. Those patients who have had no motor function for over 48 hours are unlikely to recover any useful function following treatment. If the patient has significant pain then treatment with a single fraction of 8 Gy radiotherapy should be considered for pain relief. Patients whose pain is already controlled, and who are of very poor performance status, have widespread metastases and limited life expectancy, should be discussed with their primary tumour-site clinician before considering investigation and treatment.[1]

Table 31.1 Prognostic indicators suggesting surgery is more likely to be beneficial. (See also ref.4.)

Histology (breast, prostate, multiple myeloma, lymphoma or renal cancer)
Good motor function at presentation
Good performance status
Limited comorbidity
Single-level spinal disease
Absence of visceral metastasis
Long interval from primary diagnosis

Surgery may also be considered to aid diagnosis with a biopsy, or to stabilize the unstable spine in a patient with significant instability pain. It may also be the only effective option when there is compression of the cord by bony fragments following vertebral collapse. A CT scan may sometimes assist in this decision-making process. Staging CT scans are required to gain an impression of the extent of the patient's disease, but in the context of a patient with rapid neurological deterioration clinical judgement must be used. Age is not a contraindication, but patients require careful selection as overall there is relatively less benefit to surgery and radiotherapy in the elderly. Major surgery should only be considered in those expected to live more than three months.[1] Prior radiotherapy has been considered a contraindication to surgery, with wound breakdown and infection being three times more likely than if radiotherapy is performed following surgery.[5]

The role of surgery has been addressed in a randomized controlled trial.[6] Patchell *et al.* looked at patients with single-level disease proven on MRI, good performance status and an onset of symptoms within 24 hours. They were randomized between circumferential decompressive surgery followed by radiotherapy (30 Gy in 10 fractions) and radiotherapy alone. Analysis showed a clear difference in favour of the surgical group, who were able to walk for significantly longer (median 122 days vs 13 days, $p=0.003$), had higher rates of continence, muscle strength and functional ability, and required fewer opioid analgesics and corticosteroids.

There is clear evidence that, for a select group of patients, surgery followed by radiotherapy is a beneficial treatment. However, the majority of patients presenting with MSCC have a poor prognosis, often with more extensive spinal disease and poor physiological reserve. The evidence for surgery in this group is less clear, with studies showing only modest benefit for the addition of surgery.[7] Newer surgical techniques involving percutaneous pedicle screws, cement-augmented balloon kyphoplasty, or a combination of the two, may be beneficial for this group of patients.[8] Careful patient selection is paramount. Following surgery all patients should be offered post-operative radiotherapy.

The majority of patients presenting with MSCC will be unsuitable for surgery. These patients should receive immediate radiotherapy (within 24 hours of MRI diagnosis of MSCC) as their definitive treatment. The aim of radiotherapy is to relieve compression of the spine and nerve roots by causing cell death in the rapidly dividing tumour tissue. This treatment is very effective at providing pain relief and is aimed at improving or stabilizing the neurological deficit.[1] The long-term survival of the patient is dependent upon the factors discussed previously; those patients with poor performance status, rapid deterioration, poor motor function and significant visceral disease have the poorest survival. Most patients have a limited life expectancy of only a few months, with a number of favourable patients surviving for much longer.[9] Radiotherapy schedules need to be individualized to take into account this variability in life expectancy. Studies have shown no difference in functional outcome or overall survival between schedules, but improved local control with longer treatments.[10] It is recommended that patients with a favourable prognosis should be considered for long-course treatment and those with a poor prognosis be given a single 8 Gy fraction.

If there is disease recurrence within the radiotherapy field then the options are surgery (taking into account the higher rate of wound breakdown and infection), further radiotherapy, chemotherapy, or best supportive care. Relapse immediately following radiotherapy treatment may be treated with surgery in patients who are fit enough, particularly employing newer minimally invasive surgical techniques to restrict wound size. In those who relapse locally a number of months after radiotherapy, and who remain well with good motor function, re-irradiation is a useful treatment option.[11]

Conclusion

This patient is fit and well, he retains good motor function, and urgent staging showed he has single site disease. His case demonstrates numerous factors suggestive of a good prognosis and in view of the evidence he should be considered for surgery. Surgery will relieve the spinal cord compression, stabilize the spine thus reducing pain, and allow a histological diagnosis to be made. This should be followed by palliative radiotherapy after the wound has healed. If the patient was not suitable for surgery then a biopsy should still be undertaken before treatment with palliative radiotherapy. Further systemic management will depend upon the histological diagnosis.

Further reading

1   National Institute for Health and Clinical Excellence [Internet]. *Metastatic spinal cord compression: diagnosis and management of patients at risk of or with metastatic spinal cord compression (CG75)*. London: National Institute for Health and Care Excellence. c.2013. [Issued Nov 2008, revised Oct 2012]. Available from: www.nice.org.uk/CG75

2   Graham PH, Capp A, Delaney G, *et al.* A pilot randomised comparison of dexamethasone 96 mg vs 16 mg per day for malignant spinal-cord compression treated by radiotherapy: TROG 01.05 Superdex study. *Clin Oncol* 2006; **18**: 70–6.

3   Mitera G, Loblaw A. Delays from symptom onset to treatment in malignant spinal cord compression: quantification and effect on pre-treatment neurological status. *Radiother Oncol* 2003; **69**: Abstract 141.

4   Tokuhashi Y, Matsuzaki H, Oda H, Oshima M, Junnosuke R. A revised scoring system for preoperative evaluation of metastatic spine tumour prognosis. *Spine* 2005; **30**(19): 2186–91.

5   Ghogawala Z, Mansfield F, Borges L. Spinal irradiation before surgical decompression adversely affects outcomes of surgery for symptomatic metastatic cord compression. *Spine* 2001; **26**(7): 818–24.

6   Patchell RA, Tibbs PA, Regine WF, *et al.* Direct decompressive surgical resection in the treatment of spinal cord compression caused by metastatic cancer: a randomised trial. *Lancet* 2005; **366**(9486): 643–8.

7   Rades D, Huttenlocher S, Dunst J, *et al.* Matched pair analysis comparing surgery followed by radiotherapy and radiotherapy alone for metastatic spinal cord compression. *J Clin Oncol* 2010; **28**(22): 3597–604.

8   Tancioni F, Navarria P, Pessina F, *et al.* Early surgical experience with minimally invasive percutaneous approach for patients with metastatic epidural spinal cord compression (MESCC) and poor prognoses. *Ann Surg Oncol* 2012; **19**(1): 294–300.

9   Chau LKK. Metastatic spinal cord compression: radiotherapy outcome. *J Pain Manag* 2012; **5**(1): 15–31.

10 Prewett S, Ventkitaraman R. Metastatic spinal cord compression. Review of the evidence for a dose fractionation schedule. *Clin Oncol* 2010; **22**(3): 222–30.

11 Maranzano E, Trippa F, Casale M, Anselmo P, Rossi R. Re-irradiation of metastatic spinal cord compression: definitive results of two randomized trials. *Radiother Oncol* 2011; **98**(2): 234–37.

32 Superior Vena Cava Obstruction

Chan Ton, Nabile Mohsin

Case history

A 50-year-old woman presenting with a three-month history of worsening shortness of breath, with associated cough, intermittent haemoptysis and weight loss. Computed tomography (CT) of the chest/abdomen shows a 10 × 8.5 cm superior mediastinal mass encasing local blood vessels and right main bronchus, extending to the right hilum, with a separate smaller right upper lobe nodule. Supraclavicular lymph node was palpable. Fine needle aspiration of the neck node shows small cell carcinoma. The patient re-presented as an emergency with worsening shortness of breath and neck swelling shortly after the scan and biopsy.

What are signs and symptoms of superior vena cava obstruction (SVCO)?

What is the differential diagnosis of SVCO?

What investigations would you perform in SVCO?

How would you manage SVCO?

Background

The superior vena cava (SVC) is formed from the joining of the brachiocephalic veins, and drains the upper part of the body. It is a short vein found in the upper part of the mediastinum and enters the right atrium at the level of the right hilum. A left SVC occurs in 0.3% of the population and drains into the coronary sinus. The azygos vein also joins the SVC before it enters the right atrium.

Superior vena cava obstruction (SVCO) is the complete or partial blockage of blood flow through the SVC through to the right atrium. Venous return from the head, neck and arms is thus impaired.

What are the signs and symptoms of SVCO?

Often considered an oncological emergency, SVCO is rarely immediately life-threatening, unless there has been a sudden blockage.[1] Onset can be insidious and collaterals (from the azygos vein) are formed. At the early stages there may be few signs or symptoms. Most commonly, the diagnosis is made on the clinical symptoms of facial/neck swelling and the finding of collaterals over the upper chest. Symptoms of SVCO are generally worse when the obstruction is below the entry of the azygos vein.

Table 32.1 Signs and symptoms of superior vena cava obstruction (SVCO)	
Symptoms	Signs
Breathlessness	Stridor
Hoarseness	Facial/neck/arm(s) swelling
Headaches, especially with bending or coughing	Distended neck and chest veins
Visual disturbance – blurred vision	Plethoric complexion
Dizziness	Pemberton's sign
Facial/arm swelling	Conjunctival congestion
Tiredness	Confusion

Causes of SVCO

The SVC can be compressed from an extrinsic source, or be blocked by thrombus from within the vein (Table 32.2).

SVCO was first described in syphilitic aortic aneurysms, but the aetiology has changed since the antibiotic era. Now the majority (~90%) of the causes of SVCO are malignant in origin. Lung cancer is the commonest oncological cause and accounts for about 80% of SVCO cases seen. Overall the condition is fairly rare and seen in about 4% of all lung cancers. Typically, SVCO is seen in right upper lobe and hilar cancers, and is more common in small-cell lung cancer (SCLC) than in non-small-cell lung cancer (NSCLC). In an era of increasing interventional therapeutics, non-malignant causes need to be borne in mind, especially in patients with indwelling vascular catheters.

Table 32.2 Sources of compression of superior vena cava		
	Malignant causes	Benign causes
Extrinsic compression	Lung cancer • RUL tumours • SCLC (~10%) > NSCLC (~1.7%) Mediastinal lymphadenopathy • Lymphoma • Mediastinal LN spread • Germ cell tumours Other cancers • Thymoma • Oesophageal	Non-malignant tumours • Goitre Mediastinal fibrosis • Idiopathic • Post-radiotherapy Infections • TB • Histoplasmosis Aortic aneurysm
Thrombus within SVC	Tumour invasion with clot formation	Indwelling catheters Pacemakers/defibrillators

NSCLC, non-small-cell lung cancer; RUL, right upper lobe. SCLC, small-cell lung cancer; SVC, superior vena cava; TB, tuberculosis

What investigations would you perform in SVCO?

Initial chest X-ray can be helpful, with findings that include widened superior mediastinum, widened right paratracheal stripe, right upper lobe collapse and right upper zone mass indistinct from the mediastinum. A CT scan of the thorax will outline the anatomy, and, in most cases, indicate the cause and extent of the SVCO. The investigation and management should be coordinated between acute oncology services and site specific multidisciplinary team members.

Depending upon the exact CT findings, other investigations may include: tumour markers (if germ cell tumour is suspected), bronchoscopy, mediastinoscopy (with biopsies) and venography.

Histology is important before definitive therapy, as treatment will be governed by this. Tumour biopsy may result in significant haemorrhage in the setting of SVCO. If the risk of tumour biopsy is considered high, consideration should be given to initial stenting before biopsy and definitive treatment

How would you manage malignant SVCO?

The treatment of malignant SVCO depends upon the pathology and extent of the symptoms.[2] There is currently no standard method to evaluate or grade the severity of SVCO. Initial treatment includes nursing the patient upright and the use of oxygen, dexamethasone (8–16 mg daily with PPI cover), and also low-molecular-weight heparin (LMWH) in the presence of proven thrombus. There are however, no data to support the efficacy or dosing of the steroid and LMWH in this setting. Anecdotally, diuretics have also been used with effect for the oedema associated with SVCO.

Definitive treatment involves the use of chemotherapy, radiotherapy, and more recently, vascular stents. Currently, there are only limited, mostly retrospective non-randomized trials comparing the relative efficacy of the various treatment modalities.

Chemotherapy is the treatment of choice for highly chemosensitive tumours, such as lymphoma, germ cell tumours and small cell carcinoma. Prognosis is expected to be the same as for cases without SVCO, although in SCLC the presence of SVCO often confers a slightly worse prognosis. Stenting in this setting is generally not necessary and should probably be avoided in potentially curable situations, since the long-term morbidities of stent use are unknown.

For tumours that are moderately chemosensitive or chemoresistant, such as NSCLC, radiotherapy is often the treatment of choice. In patients with significant symptoms, stenting may be more appropriate in the first instance to alleviate the effects of SVCO.

Vascular stenting is the placement of an endovascular tube to re-canalize the SVC and re-establish blood flow. Stents are placed percutaneously with radiological guidance and following caval venography plus/minus clot lysis. The limited data on stent use suggest rapid improvement of SVCO symptoms in most lung cancer patients (often 1–3 days), relatively lower risk of re-blockage, and longer duration of patency.[3,4] Overall survival seems unaffected. At present, it is uncertain whether long-term anticoagulation is necessary following stent insertion. Generally, the procedure is minimally invasive, well tolerated and fairly safe. Complications have been reported, including stent migration and thrombosis, venous tear, cardiac tamponade, acute cardiogenic pulmonary oedema and pain, but these are rare. Re-stenting has been reported to be feasible and successful.

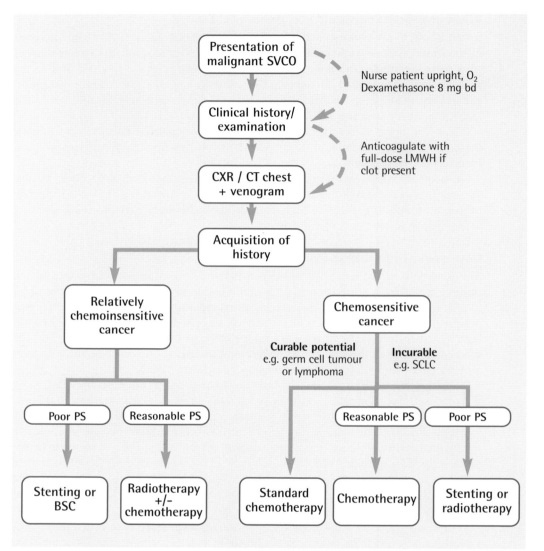

Figure 32.1 Suggested management of superior vena cava obstruction (SVCO). CT, computed tomography; CXR, chest X-ray; PS, performance status.

Stent insertion has, in the past, mostly been used after the failure of chemotherapy or radiotherapy. However, given that it provides rapid relief of symptoms with minimal complications, stenting may now need to be considered for use as a first definitive treatment in the palliative setting. The normal oncological therapies may follow. There is, however, a noticeable lack of prospective data to compare the use of stents with chemotherapy and radiotherapy, and how quality of life might be different with each modality. The Cochrane Review data presented by Rowel and Geeson,[5] where most trials were non-randomized, suggested that for all lung cancers stenting provides relief of SVCO symptoms in 95% of patients, with a relapse rate of 11%. For SCLC, chemotherapy with/without radiotherapy achieved 77% response rate with 17% relapsed, and for NSCLC the response rate was 60% with a relapse rate of 19%. Furthermore, symptomatic relief was more rapid with stenting.

Conclusions

SVCO is generally a rare oncological presentation. It is most commonly seen in right-sided lung cancer and is generally not life-threatening. The treatment of SVCO and its prognosis are determined by the exact causal pathology.

Vascular stenting appears to confer rapid relief of SVCO symptoms and should be considered as part of the treatment armamenum. However, data are lacking on the best time for its use.

Further reading

1   Schraufnagel DE, Hill R Leech JA, Pare JA. Superior vena cava obstruction: Is it a medical emergency? *Am J Med* 1981; **70**: 1169–74.

2   Saadeen A, Abdul-Rahman J. Management of lung cancer-related complications. *Ann Thorac Med* 2008; **6**: 104–7.

3   Greillier L, Barlesi F, Doddoli C, *et al.* Vascular stenting for palliation of superior vena cava obstruction in non-small-cell lung cancer patients: a future 'standard' procedure? *Respiration* 2004; **71**: 178–83.

4   Nicholson AA, Ettles DF, Arnold A, Greenstone M, Dyet JF. Treatment of malignant superior vena cava: metal stents or radiation therapy. *J Vasc Intervent Radiol* 1997; **8**: 781–8.

5   Rowell NP, Geeson FV. Steroids, radiotherapy, chemotherapy and stents for superior veno caval obstruction in carcinoma of the bronchus. *Cochrane Database Syst Rev* 2001; **4**: CD001316.

33 Brain Metastases

Pooja Jain, Allison Hall, Andrew Brodbelt

Case history

A 54-year-old male smoker presents with a five-day history of expressive dysphasia and a 24-hour history of confusion and headache. He has no other neurological symptoms or signs and is otherwise fit and well. A brain computed tomography (CT) scan shows multiple ring-enhancing lesions in both cerebral hemispheres surrounded by marked oedema. The oedema is causing 11 mm of midline shift. Appearances are consistent with multiple brain metastases (Figure 33.1).

What is the immediate management of this patient?

What investigations does the patient need?

What is the definitive management of this patient?

Background

Brain metastases affect 20%–40% of patients with malignancy during the course of their illness and cause significant morbidity even with treatment. A suggested management pathway is illustrated in Figure 33.2. The most common primary tumours sites are lung (44%), breast (15%), renal (7%) and melanoma (7%). Presenting symptoms include headache (49%), focal weakness (30%), gait ataxia (21%) and seizures (18%).

Prognosis following a diagnosis of brain metastases is poor, with a median survival of 1–2 months. With treatment, prognosis may be improved but patients must be carefully selected to prevent unnecessary toxicity in the last few weeks of life. Various prognostic indices can be used to help guide appropriate management, as a patient with a solitary brain metastasis is likely to have differing outcomes and management than someone with multiple metastases.[1] Recursive partitioning analysis (RPA), a study which combined data from three North American trials, can be used to predict patients likely to benefit from therapy.[2] The RPA score categorizes patients into three groups based on the Karnofsky performance scale, primary tumour status, age and the presence of extracranial disease (Table 33.1).

Other factors, such as primary site of disease and number of metastases, are important as they may also dictate prognosis.[3] Patients with breast cancer primaries and those patients with fewer metastases do better. Treatment for brain metastases is predominantly with corticosteroids and whole-brain radiotherapy. Patients with solitary or oligometastases should be considered for local treatment with surgery or stereotactic radiosurgery (SRS).[4–6]

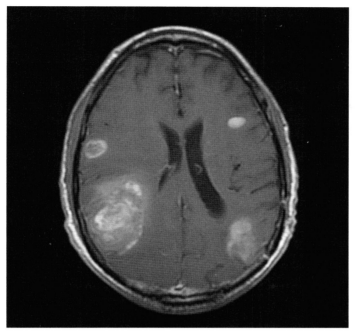

Figure 33.1 Brain CT scan with contrast showing multiple enhancing brain metastases with surrounding vasogenic oedema and effacement of the ventricle.

Table 33.1 Prognostic groups for outcome after palliative radiotherapy of brain metastases by recursive partitioning analysis (see also ref.2).

Class	Prognostic factors	Median survival, months
I	KPS >70%	7.1
	Age <65 years	
	Controlled primary site	
	No extracranial metastases	
II	KPS < 70	2.3
III	All others	4.2

KPS, Karnofsky score for performance status.

What is the immediate management of this patient?

High-dose dexamethasone reduces cerebral oedema. This provides symptomatic relief and may produce improved function and quality of life. A typical regimen is dexamethasone 16 mg daily for 48 h followed by gradual reduction to a maintenance dose of 2–4 mg daily. Without a reducing regimen, high doses of corticosteroids have potentially debilitating neuromuscular, psychological, cosmetic, gastrointestinal and metabolic side effects. Hyperglycaemia and confusion can be particular difficult to control. Prophylactic gastric cover should be considered using proton pump inhibitors.

Patients presenting with seizure activity should be offered anticonvulsant therapy according to local policy and to prevent further episodes. For those with complex symptom control, early involvement of specialist palliative care is beneficial.

What investigations does the patient need?

Intensity of investigations must be appropriate to the prognosis of the patient. Performance status of the patient is a key driver of investigations as this also dictates management and outcome for the patient.[7] Specialist advice should be sought to avoid procedures and imaging that are unlikely to alter management in order to prevent unnecessary discomfort and distress.

For lesions that are suspected to be solitary on contrast-enhanced CT, magnetic resonance imaging (MRI) with gadolinium is indicated to assess the extent of intracranial disease and resectability. Malignant differential diagnosis of a solitary intracranial lesion includes:

- solitary metastasis from an extracranial primary tumour
- primary brain tumour
- primary central nervous system (CNS) lymphoma
- cerebral abscess.

Extracranial disease is assessed by CT. In patients with known malignancy, this establishes the status of disease as either progressive or stable. In those with their first presentation of malignancy, the management should follow the steps outlined for suspected malignancy of unknown origin.

An acute oncology service can facilitate multidisciplinary involvement of neurosurgeons, radiologists, oncologists and pathologists to ensure the prompt and appropriate management of brain metastases.

Role of surgery

There are 3 main indications for surgery:

1. Resection of solitary or few (usually ≤3) accessible metastases
2. Palliation of hydrocephalus/debulking of large metastases
3. Biopsy for histological diagnosis.

1. Resection of a solitary or few (usually ≤3) accessible metastases

Neurosurgery should be considered for patients of reasonable performance status either before or following steroid loading, or in those for whom surgery will improve their performance status score. The risk of complications should be acceptably low and extracranial disease controlled.

Overall, local and distal cerebral recurrence rates are improved by following resection with whole-brain radiotherapy (WBRT).[8]

2. Palliation of hydrocephalus/debulking of large metastases

Surgical decompression relieves symptoms of raised intracranial pressure. Radiotherapy has limited benefit for large (>5 cm), cystic, or cerebellar lesions – therefore, it is reasonable to resect such lesions if symptomatic. The risk of complications must be acceptable to both surgeon and patient.

Figure 33.2 Management of suspected brain metastases

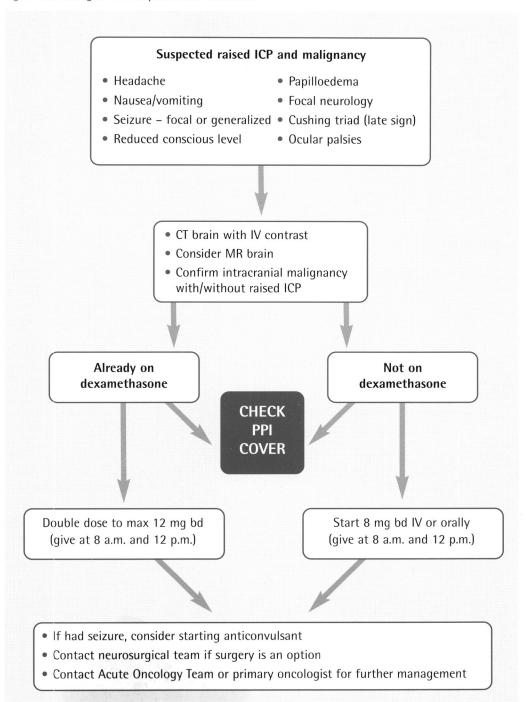

3. Biopsy for histological diagnosis

Histological diagnosis is of benefit to patients fit enough to be considered for systemic treatment. In the absence of a more accessible lesion amenable to endoscopic or percutaneous biopsy, this procedure can aid both diagnosis and estimation of prognosis. Ten per cent of patients presenting with a brain metastasis will have no identifiable primary tumour.

Role of radiotherapy

Whole-brain radiotherapy (WBRT) remains the accepted standard treatment for palliation of brain metastases.[9] However, aggressive local palliation with combinations of SRS and surgery are becoming more popular. Exceptions to radiotherapeutic treatments are tumours with high intrinsic chemosensitivity, e.g. lymphoma or germ cell tumours. Patients with metastases suitable for resection or SRS should be referred for a neurosurgical opinion.

Common toxicities of WBRT include fatigue, alopecia, scalp erythema and impaired higher cognitive function. More unusual side effects are somnolence syndrome and severe headaches.

Recently, the role of WBRT for treatment of brain metastases from solid malignancies (except chemosensitive cancers) has been questioned, particularly with reference to limited symptomatic gain, quality of life and undue toxicity at the end of life.[10] This is the subject of a UK randomized trial (QUARTZ) that is evaluating WBRT in the management of brain metastases in non-small-cell lung cancer.

Relapse

Almost without exception, intracranial relapse is rapidly fatal. For a minority of patients with oligometastases, resection or SRS may offer disease control and better prognosis. Symptomatic treatment with corticosteroids is often the only intervention.

For patients who maintain good performance status despite relapse, systemic cytotoxic therapy and emerging biological targeted therapies remain an option in selected cases.

Stereotactic radiosurgery (SRS)

Stereotactic radiosurgery includes Gamma Knife and linear particle accelerator-based systems that deliver high-dose radiotherapy with millimetre accuracy to a sharply defined target, largely sparing the surrounding normal tissue, with the patient often admitted as a day case. Strict criteria are necessary to ensure appropriate patient selection. Common selection criteria include up to four metastases ≤4 cm, in patients with controlled or only slowly progressing distal disease that does not require surgery for mass effect, obstructed cerebrospinal fluid flow, or diagnosis.

The question of whether SRS is equivalent to surgery is unanswered, with studies producing conflicting results and no good randomized controlled trials. The data so far suggest that SRS is equivalent to surgery for tumour control, but with fewer risks. The choice of SRS over surgery is often based on surgical accessibility, size of the lesion, functional status of the patient, and the local availability of SRS.[11,12]

Conclusion

Brain metastases usually herald a poor prognosis for most cancer patients. Most patients with brain metastases routinely receive dexamethasone either as sole treatment or in addition to WBRT. The performance status of a patient, primary site, number of metastases and control of extracranial disease are important determinators of appropriate management and eventual outcome. Patients with ≤3 metastases can benefit from aggressive management and should be discussed promptly with the regional neurosurgical service.

Further reading

1   Barnholtz-Sloan JS, Yu C, Sloan AE, *et al.* A nomogram for individualized estimation of survival among patients with brain metastasis. *Neuro Oncol* 2012; **14**(7): 910–8.

2   Gaspar L, Scott C, Rotman M, *et al.* Recursive partitioning analysis (RPA) of prognostic factors in three Radiation Therapy Oncology Group (RTOG) brain metastases trials. *Int J Radiat Oncol Biol Phys* 1997; **37**(4): 745–51.

3   Sperduto PW, Chao ST, Sneed PK, *et al.* Diagnosis-specific prognostic factors, indexes, and treatment outcomes for patients with newly diagnosed brain metastases: a multi-institutional analysis of 4,259 patients. *Int J Radiat Oncol Biol Phys* 2010; **77**: 655–61.

4   Andrews DW, Scott CB, Sperduto PW, *et al.* Whole brain radiation therapy with or without stereotactic radiosurgery boost for patients with one to three brain metastases: phase III results of the RTOG 9508 randomised trial. *Lancet* 2004; **363**(9422): 1665–72.

5   Gates M, Alsaidi M, Kalkanis S. Surgical treatment of solitary brain metastases. *Prog Neurol Surg* 2012; **25**: 74–81.

6   Niranjan A, Lunsford LD, Emerick RL. Stereotactic radiosurgery for patients with metastatic brain tumors: development of a consensus radiosurgery guideline recommendation. *Prog Neurol Surg* 2012; **25**: 123–38.

7   Tsao MN, Lloyd NS, Wong RK. Clinical practice guideline on the optimal radiotherapeutic management of brain metastases. *BMC Cancer* 2005; **5**: 34.

8   Patchell RA, Tibbs PA, Walsh JW, *et al.* A randomized trial of surgery in the treatment of single metastases to the brain. *N Engl J Med* 1990; **322**(8): 494–500.

9   Tsao MN, Lloyd N, Wong RK, *et al.* Whole brain radiotherapy for the treatment of multiple brain metastases. *Cochrane Database Syst Rev* 2012; **4**: CD003869.

10   Bezjak A, Adam J, Barton R, *et al.* Symptom response after palliative radiotherapy for patients with brain metastases. *Eur J Cancer* 2002; **38**(4): 487–96.

11   Auchter RM, Lamond JP, Alexander E, *et al.* A multiinstitutional outcome and prognostic factor analysis of radiosurgery for resectable single brain metastasis. *Int J Radiat Oncol Biol Phys* 1996; **35**(1): 27–35.

12   Bindal AK, Bindal RK, Hess KR, *et al.* Surgery versus radiosurgery in the treatment of brain metastasis. *J Neurosurg* 1996; **84**(5): 748–54.

PROBLEM

34 Paraneoplastic Syndromes

Greg Heath, Susan Short, Helen Ford

Case history

A 65-year-old woman with stage II ovarian cancer and hypothyroidism is admitted onto the acute oncology ward with a five-day history of progressive nausea, gait instability and oscillopsia. The patient does not drink alcohol and her only medication is thyroxine replacement therapy. On examination she manifests a downbeat nystagmus, past pointing, dysdiadochokinesia, and both truncal and gait ataxia.

What is the differential diagnosis?

What investigations would you do or request?

What is the treatment and prognosis?

Background

What is the differential diagnosis?

The signs and symptoms are suggestive of a cerebellar lesion. In the context of a person with a known malignancy, cerebellar metastases and paraneoplastic syndromes would be high on your list of differentials. Other conditions to consider include vascular (infarction/ischaemia), metabolic causes, medications (for example anticonvulsants) and thyroid dysfunction. In the context of patients with known cancer, practitioners should be cognisant of cerebellar insults secondary to certain types of chemotherapy, such as cytarabine and fluorouracil.

What investigations would you request?

Urgent neuroimaging is required to exclude a cerebellar mass. Magnetic resonance imaging (MRI) is more sensitive than computed tomography (CT) in detecting lesions within the cerebellum and brainstem, and should be requested if the initial CT scan is negative. Routine blood tests, including thyroid function, should be taken. Hypothyroidism is a rare, albeit treatable, cause of cerebellar dysfunction. Vitamin B and E levels should also be measured because deficiencies may interfere with cerebellar function.

Both the laboratory and radiological investigations fail to reveal an abnormality to explain the patient's cerebellar signs and symptoms.

What is the most likely diagnosis?

The most likely diagnosis is a paraneoplastic syndrome affecting the cerebellum, in particular paraneoplastic cerebellar degeneration (PCD). As a consequence, paraneoplastic biomarkers should be measured in the patient's serum.

What are paraneoplastic syndromes?

By definition, paraneoplastic syndromes are a heterogeneous group of neurological disorders that are associated with systemic cancer, but not by the cancer *per se* or side effects of its treatment. Although not completely understood, it is conjectured that these syndromes arise as result of an immunological response directed against shared antigens (in particular the nervous system) that are ectopically released by the tumour.[1] A suggestion has been made that self-antigens may be processed differently in cancer cells, thus inciting a T-cell response.[2]

It is noteworthy that paraneoplastic syndromes may arise from a non-immune, pathophysiological basis. An example is the release of hormones by a tumour, such as parathyroid hormone-related peptide (PTHrP) leading to hypercalcaemia.

Numerous onconeural antibodies have been identified. Antibodies that have been classified as 'well characterized' are summarized in Table 34.1. The presence of any of these antibodies in a patient's serum is sufficient to define them as harbouring a paraneoplastic syndrome even in the absence of detecting an underlying neoplasia.[3] Patients harbouring 'partially characterized antibodies', by contrast, require a diagnosis of cancer in order to be diagnosed as suffering from a paraneoplastic syndrome. Examples of these antibodies are illustrated in Table 34.2.

Table 34.1 Well-characterized paraneoplastic antibodies

Antibody	Syndrome	Associated Cancer
Anti-Yo (PCA-1)	Cerebellar degeneration	Ovarian, breast
Anti-Hu (ANNA-1)	Cerebellar degeneration, limbic, brainstem encephalitis, sensory neuropathy	SCLC
Anti-amphiphysin	Stiff person syndrome, encephalomyelitis	Breast, lung cancer
Anti-CRMP5 (CV2)	Encephalomyelitis, cerebellar degeneration, peripheral neuropathy	SCLC, thymoma
Anti-Tr	Cerebellar degeneration	Hodgkin lymphoma
Anti-Ri (ANNA-2)	Cerebellar degeneration, brainstem encephalitis, opsoclonus-myoclonus	Breast, gynaecological, SCLC
Anti-recoverin	Cancer-associated retinopathy	SCLC
Anti-Ma proteins	Limbic or brainstem encephalitis	Germ cell tumours, lung cancer

ANNA, anti-neuronal nuclear antibody; CRMP, collapsin response mediator protein; PCA, Purkinje cell antibody; SCLC, small-cell lung cancer.

Table 34.2 **Partially characterized paraneoplastic antibodies**		
Antibody	Syndrome	Associated Cancers
ANNA-3	Sensory neuropathy, enecephalomyelitis	SCLC
PCA-2	Encephalomyelitis, cerebellar degeneration	SCLC
Anti-Zic 4	Cerebellar degeneration	SCLC
mGluR1	Cerebellar degeneration	Hodgkin lymphoma
Anti-bipolar retinal cells	Melanoma-associated retinopathy	Melanoma

ANNA, antineuronal nuclear antibody; mGluR1, metabotropic glutamate receptor 1; PCA, Purkinje cell antibody; SCLC, small-cell lung cancer.

As one can see from the list of antibodies in Tables 34.1 and 34.2, the cerebellum is a frequent target of paraneoplastic autoimmunity. Relevant to this case, the anti-Yo antibody is predominantly associated with cerebellar degeneration as a result of ovarian cancer.[4]

Although paraneoplastic antibodies may be detected in the patient's cerebrospinal fluid (CSF) and therefore provide confirmatory evidence of the existence of a paraneoplastic disorder, they are usually present in the serum as well.[5] In patients with coexisting encephalitis, lumbar puncture is useful to ascertain whether the signs and symptoms are secondary to leptomeningeal carcinomatosis, or if they are immune-mediated. The presence of malignant cells is highly indicative of the former, whereas identification of oligoclonal bands, intrathecal synthesis of IgG, and/or a mild pleocytosis (10–50 lymphocytes) is suggestive of the latter.

As in this case, MRI frequently fails to elicit any abnormality in the acute setting in patients suffering from paraneoplastic cerebellar degeneration. Occasionally, one may find enhancement with gadolinium within the cerebellum or generalized atrophy in the chronic phase.[6]

What is the treatment and prognosis?

 The patient's serum is positive for anti-Yo antibodies, thus providing confirmatory evidence of paraneoplastic cerebellar degeneration.

Unfortunately, the outcome is usually poor. The majority of patients either become or remain non-ambulatory.[7] It is worthy of note that the antibody type may be of value prognostically. Anti-Yo antibodies are associated with a less favourable outcome (median survival of 13 months) than its Hodgkin lymphoma-associated counterpart, anti-Tr (median survival 113 months).[7] Advancing age and progression of the patient's underlying cancer also correlate positively with increased morbidity and mortality.

Treatment of the underlying tumour is essential in attempting to stabilize or ameliorate the neurological sequelae. Intuitively, immunotherapy should improve the patient's symptoms. In practice it has been met with negative results.[7] Notwithstanding, anecdotal reports exist extolling the virtues of immunosuppressant agents such as corticosteroids and rituximab.[8] A case report and concomitant literature review illuminated the potential benefits of administering intravenous immunoglobulin within three months of the onset of symptoms.[9] As a result, there is a cogent argument to suggest such therapy if paraneoplastic cerebellar degeneration is detected within the aforementioned time period.

Conclusion

The presence of neurological signs and symptoms in a patient with a known oncological diagnosis and negative neuroimaging should alert practitioners to the possibility of a coexisting paraneoplastic syndrome. Serum antibodies may support the diagnosis. Cerebrospinal fluid antibodies are not always necessary, but analysis of CSF may aid the practitioner in cases where diagnosis is difficult. Treatment of the underlying cancer is essential before considering immunotherapy. Paraneoplastic syndromes associated with well-characterized antibodies confer a worse prognosis.

Further reading

1 Dalmau J, Gultekin HS, Posner JB. Paraneoplastic neurologic syndromes: pathogenesis and physiopathology. *Brain Pathol* 1999; **9**: 275.

2 Savage PA, Vosseller K, Kang C, *et al.* Recognition of a ubiquitous self antigen by prostate cancer-infiltrating CD8+ T lymphocytes. *Science* 2008; **319**: 215–20.

3 Graus F, Delattre JY, Antoine JC, *et al.* Recommended diagnostic criteria for paraneoplastic neurological syndromes. *J Neurol Neurosurg Psychiatry* 2004; **75**: 1135–40.

4 McKeon A, Tracey JA, Pittock SJ, *et al.* Purkinje cell cytoplasmic autoantibody type 1 accompaniments: the cerebellum and beyond. *Arch Neurol* 2011; **68**(10): 1282–9.

5 McKeon A, Pittock SJ, Lennon VA. CSF complements serum for evaluating paraneoplastic antibodies and NMO-IgG. *Neurology* 2011; **76**(12): 1108–10.

6 Gozzard P, Maddison P. Which antibody and which cancer in which paraneoplastic syndromes? *Pract Neurol* 2010; **10**: 260–70.

7 Shams'ili S, Grefkens J, de Leeuw B, *et al.* Paraneoplastic cerebellar degeneration associated with antineuronal antibodies: analysis of 50 patients. *Brain* 2003; **126**: 1409–18.

8 Esposito M, Penza P, Orefice G, *et al.* Successful treatment of paraneoplastic cerebellar degeneration with rituximab. *J Neurooncol* 2008; **8**(3): 363–4.

9 Widdess-Walsh P, Tavee JO, Schuele S, Stevens GH. Response to intravenous immunoglobulin in anti-Yo associated paraneoplastic cerebellar degeneration: a case report and a review of the literature. *J Neurooncol* 2003; **63**(2): 187–90.

PROBLEM

35 Venous Thromboembolism

Anna Mullard, Helen Innes, Maged Gharib

Case history

A 68-year-old man receiving palliative chemotherapy for metastatic pancreatic carcinoma is admitted to the acute medical assessment unit complaining of dyspnoea and pleuritic chest pain. He undergoes a CT pulmonary angiogram (CTPA) which confirms a pulmonary embolism (Figure 35.1).

Why did this occur?

What is the optimal management of this patient?

Should this patient be managed differently if this were an incidental finding?

What should be done if the patient develops a further embolic event while on treatment?

Could this have been prevented?

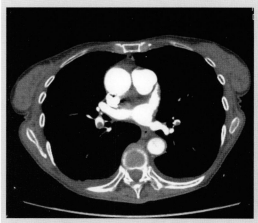 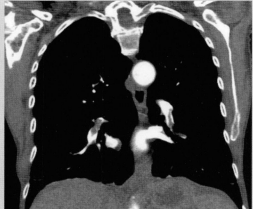

Figure 35.1 Axial and coronal CTPA images showing right lower lobe pulmonary embolism

Background

Why did this occur?

Venous thromboembolism (VTE) is an important cause of morbidity and mortality in patients with cancer. It occurs in up to 20% of patients with an overt malignancy and is the second leading cause of death in these patients.[1] Consequently, a low threshold for investigating suggestive signs or symptoms should be adopted in any cancer patient.

Clinicians must also be aware of the possibility of atypical presentation of VTE in patients with cancer (such as a more gradual increasing breathlessness), which may be due to symptom masking by the underlying malignant disease and/or its treatment.

Given the high risk, it is not surprising that a VTE may even precede the diagnosis of cancer. Current guidance suggests investigating all patients over the age of 40 years with an unprovoked first VTE for the possibility of an occult malignancy.[2]

Virchow's triad suggests that VTE occurs due to three factors: alteration in blood flow, vascular endothelial injury, and alteration in the constituents of the blood. All of these implicating factors may be seen in malignancy. Turbulent blood flow can occur due to extrinsic compression from malignant tumours, or intrinsic devices such as central venous catheters. Vascular endothelial injury can be induced by systemic anticancer therapies – some of the newer agents, such as angiogenesis inhibitors, are known to confer a particularly high risk. A hypercoagulable state may be induced by malignancy, whereby both tumour and normal cells produce procoagulant agents. Deep vein thrombosis (DVT) and pulmonary embolus (PE) are the most common form of VTE, but other forms, e.g. migratory superficial thrombophlebitis (Trosseau's syndrome), disseminated intravascular coagulation, thrombotic microangiopathy and arterial thrombosis, are also known to be more common in patients with cancer.

In addition to advanced disease, certain types of cancer are known to afford a particularly high risk for VTE, including: pancreatic, bladder, gastric, uterine, kidney and lung cancers. Patients undergoing systemic anticancer treatment have a 7-fold increased risk of VTE.[3] Many of the other risk factors for VTE are also common features in cancer patients (Table 35.1).

Table 35.1 Risk factors for venous thromboembolism (VTE) in patients with malignant disease. (Adapted from ref. 1.)

Cancer related
Primary site of cancer – pancreatic, gastric, uterine, kidney, lung
Extensive disease
Initial 3-6 months after diagnosis
Active systemic anticancer therapy including hormone therapy and anti-angiogenic therapy
Presence of central venous catheter
Recent steroid therapy
Recent major surgery
Prolonged hospitalization

Other
Older age
Raised body mass index
Prior history of VTE
Reduced mobility
Ethnicity (increased in those of black African descent)

What is the optimal management of this patient?

Where possible, treatment of a VTE in a cancer patient should be with low-molecular-weight heparin (LMWH) for a minimum of six months. Oral anticoagulation is less effective in preventing further VTE.[4] However, oral anticoagulation does not significantly increase bleeding rate or diminish survival compared to LMWH and, therefore, remains an option in patients who find daily injections unacceptable.[4] Fluctuating INR levels as a result of cancer-related factors (e.g. malnutrition, liver dysfunction and drug interactions) are some of the probable causes of decreased efficacy of oral anticoagulation in this group of patients. A variety of LMWHs are used in the treatment of VTE, but it should be noted that to date dalteparin is the only drug licensed for extended use in oncology patients.

Relative contraindications to LMWH include recent haemorrhage, active gastric/duodenal ulcer, acute bacterial endocarditis and thrombocytopenia; many clinicians would not anticoagulate patients with a platelet count of <50. Any patient with these issues may be considered for inferior vena cava (IVC) filter until the contraindication has resolved, at which point LMWH should be initiated in addition to the filter.[2]

Patients with severe renal impairment, i.e. estimated GFR <30 ml/min, should be treated with unfractionated heparin.[2] However, continued treatment with reduced-dose LMWH and monitoring of anti-factor Xa may be more convenient if the renal function is unlikely to improve.

Although data are lacking regarding LMWH treatment beyond six months, consensus opinion is that prophylactic LMWH dose should continue indefinitely as long as there is clinical evidence of active malignant disease and the benefit outweighs the risk.[3]

Any patient with haemodynamic instability as a result of either PE, or extensive DVT causing risk to limb perfusion, should be considered for thrombolytic therapy in addition to anticoagulation. However, the potential risks and benefits to the individual patient must be carefully considered.

Should this patient be managed differently if this were an incidental finding?

The increased use of high-resolution CT scans for disease assessment in patients with cancer has led to the diagnosis of incidental PE becoming a common clinical scenario. Although management of VTE is based on data from symptomatic patients, it is widely accepted that these patients with asymptomatic PE require prompt assessment and initiation of anticoagulation in the same way.

Treatment of these patients may present logistical problems, since the diagnosis of VTE may be made while they are in the radiology department or after they have left the hospital premises. Many experienced clinicians routinely initiate outpatient anticoagulation in such patients. However, there are no validated criteria to define patient groups for whom this is safe or whether admission is appropriate. Outpatient management of DVT (and possibly PE) appears to be a viable option for selected patients, and should be considered if supportive services are in place. Development of robust pathways integrating radiology, acute oncology and acute medical departments is necessary to standardize and streamline the management for these patients.

What should be done if the patient develops a further embolic event while on treatment?

A small proportion of patients will go on to have a further VTE despite anticoagulation: 9% of patients on LMWH and 17% of patients on oral anticoagulation.[4] For those who have had suboptimal treatment in the form of missed doses, efforts to optimize treatment should be undertaken. Patients on oral anticoagulation should be switched to LMWH where possible. Patients having recurrent VTE despite optimal therapy should be considered for IVC filter placement.[2] Twice-daily LMWH regimens are advisable in these patients (enoxaparin 1 mg/kg twice-daily instead of 1.5 mg/kg once daily) with pre- and 3–4 h post-dose anti-Xa activity monitoring.

Could this have been prevented?

Although patients with malignancy are known to have higher risk of VTE, for those who are ambulatory there are insufficient data to support the use of primary prophylaxis. Several randomized trials have found a clear reduction in VTE in ambulant patients undergoing chemotherapy with LMWH, but have thus far failed to show an overall survival advantage.[5–8] An important unanswered question is whether it might be possible to define any high-risk group(s) in whom primary VTE prophylaxis would confer a survival advantage.

For immobile patients with cancer, such as those admitted to hospital or those undergoing a surgical procedure, the rate of VTE is over 30% and thus prophylactic LMWH is recommended.[3] It is appropriate to omit VTE prophylaxis in patients admitted to hospital for terminal care.[9]

Conclusion

VTE is an important cause of morbidity and mortality in cancer patients. Patients diagnosed with a thromboembolic event should receive prompt treatment with LMWH, and this should ideally continue long-term rather than switching to an oral anticoagulant. Despite optimal treatment for a VTE, a minority of cancer patients will go on to have further events requiring consideration for an IVC filter.

Although patients with cancer are known to be at increased risk of VTE, primary prophylaxis is not routinely recommended unless the patient is immobilized or is undergoing a surgical procedure.

Further reading

1   Lyman GH, Khorana AA, Falanga A, *et al.* American Society of Clinical Oncology Guideline: recommendations for venous thromboembolism prophylaxis and treatment in patients with cancer. *J Clin Oncol* 2007; **25**(34): 5490–505.

2   National Institute for Health and Clinical Excellence. *Venous thromboembolic diseases: the management of venous thromboembolic diseases and the role of thrombophilia testing.* CG144. [Issued Jun 2012]. London: National Institute for Health and Care Excellence. c.2012.

3   Mandala M, Falanga A, Roila F. Management of venous thromboembolism (VTE) in cancer patients: ESMO Clinical Practice Guidelines. *Ann Oncol* 2011; **22**(supplement 6): vi85–vi92.

4   Lee AY, Levine MN, Baker RI, *et al.*; Randomized Comparison of Low-Molecular-Weight Heparin Versus Oral Anticoagulant Therapy for the Prevention of Recurrent Venous Thromboembolism in Patients with Cancer (CLOT) Investigators. Low-molecular-weight heparin versus a coumarin for the prevention of recurrent venous thromboembolism in patients with cancer. *N Engl J Med* 2003; **349**: 146–53.

5   Agnelli G, Gussoni G, Bianchini C, *et al.* Nadroparin for the prevention of thromboembolic events in ambulatory patients with metastatic or locally advanced solid cancer receiving chemotherapy: a randomised, placebo-controlled, double blind study. *Lancet Oncol* 2009; **10**(10): 943–9.

6   Riess H, Pelzer U, Deutschinoff G, *et al.* A prospective, randomised trial of chemotherapy with or without the low molecular weight hepain (LMWH) enoxaparin in patients with advanced pancreatic cancer: Results of the CONKO 004 trial [Abstract]. *J Clin Oncol* 2009: **27**: 798s.

7   Maraveyas A, Waters J, Roy R, *et al.* Gemcitabine versus gemcitabine plus dalteparin in pancreatic cancer. *Eur J Cancer* 2012; **48**(9): 1283–92.

8   Agnelli G, George DJ, Kakkar AK, *et al.* Semuloparin for thromboprophylaxis in patients receiving chemotherapy for cancer. *N Engl J Med* 2012; **366**(7): 601–9.

9   National Institute for Health and Clinical Excellence. *Reducing the risk of venous thromboembolism (deep vein thrombosis and pulmonary embolus) in patients admitted to hospital.* CG92. [Issued Jan 2010]. London: National Institute for Health and Care Excellence. c.2010.

36 Malignant Renal Obstruction

Shaker Abdallah, Jonathan Wide

Case history

A 60-year-old woman with known advanced ovarian cancer presents to the emergency department with abdominal swelling associated with nausea and constipation. The patient had previously undergone extensive surgery and multiple lines of chemotherapy. A blood test on admission revealed impaired renal function with a serum creatinine of 280 μmol/l. Abdominal ultrasound revealed bilateral hydronephrosis.

What is the differential diagnosis?

How would you investigate the patient?

How would you manage this patient?

Background

Malignant obstructive uropathy occurs when obstruction of the urine flow due to malignant infiltration, or external compression of the urinary tract in the retroperitoneum or pelvis, results in increased collecting system pressure, urinary stasis and renal failure. The obstruction can be partial or complete, unilateral or bilateral, and it can occur at any level below or above the bladder.

Obstruction of the urinary tract may result from a range of primary malignancies (Table 36.1) or occasionally represent a late complication of external beam radiotherapy to the abdomen and pelvis.[1] Extrinsic obstruction may be due to direct compression or encasement of the urinary tract by retroperitoneal tumour or malignant lymphadenopathy, or invasion of the ureter, bladder neck or urethra by the primary or metastatic cancer.[2–4] Gynaecological and urological cancers are the most common causes, followed by gastrointestinal and other sites, including metastatic breast cancer or lymphoma. Prostate cancer is the most common cause in males, whereas uterine cervix cancer is the most common cause in females.

Intrinsic obstruction is caused by transitional cell carcinoma of the bladder, renal pelvis or ureter.

Table 36.1 Most common causes of malignant obstructive uropathy
Uterine cervix and endometrial cancer
Bladder cancer
Prostate cancer
Colorectal cancer
Ovarian cancer
Lymphoma

Symptoms and signs

Symptoms may vary depending on the site of obstruction (upper or lower), the degree, the speed of onset and whether it is unilateral or bilateral. Malignant obstruction typically develops over a long period of time causing minimal or no symptoms, and is frequently discovered on routine imaging performed for staging purposes or triggered by abnormal renal function on routine blood test.

Both partial and complete obstruction increase the tendency for urinary tract infections, which may present with acute clinical deterioration and systemic sepsis.

Rectal or pelvic examination can reveal rectal, prostate or uterine cervix tumours as possible causes of urinary obstruction. General examination may detect increased abdominal girth due to the underlying cancer, enlarged kidney, bladder or palpable abdominopelvic mass. Further clinical signs include, volume overload, weight gain and bilateral leg oedema.

Differential diagnosis

The patient presents with advanced intra-abdominal malignancy following multiple lines of potentially nephrotoxic drugs. Possible diagnoses include: intrinsic renal impairment; malignant bowel obstruction; malignant ascites; prerenal impairment secondary to nausea and reduced oral intake; bladder retention secondary to pelvic infiltration; hydronephrosis secondary to malignant ureteric obstruction; or a combination of all of these factors.

How would you manage the patient?

The management of patients with advanced abdominopelvic malignancy presenting with renal obstruction as a result of the underlying cancer depends on various factors, including patient fitness, degree of renal obstruction, the outlook of the underlying disease and whether further effective treatment is available (Figure 36.1). An aggressive approach to decompress the kidneys is indicated if the patient remains with good performance status, particularly if further effective treatment is still available and in the setting of acute urosepsis. Best supportive care with symptomatic measures should be considered if the patient's general condition is poor, and/or further anticancer treatment is not expected to have any meaningful impact on the natural behaviour of the cancer and patient's quality of life.

Diagnosis

The level and cause of obstruction should be identified before making the appropriate management decisions. Abdominal ultrasound is non-invasive and readily available, and in this case revealed a small amount of ascites and bilateral hydronephrosis. Intravenous

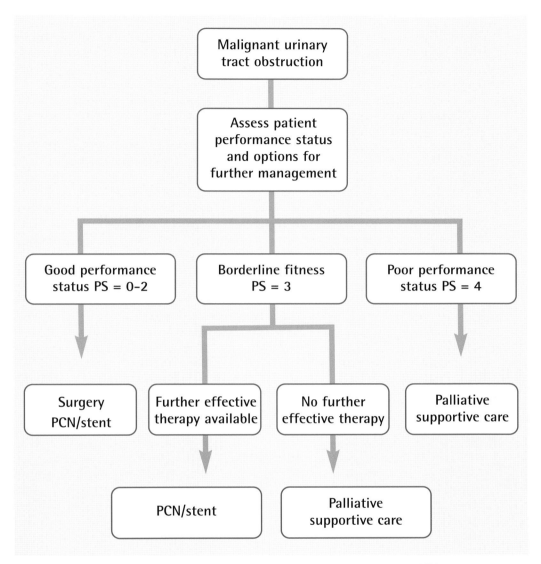

Figure 36.1 Algorithm for managing urinary tract obstruction in advanced cancer patients. PCN, percutaneous nephrostomy.

contrast enhancement is a relative contraindication in the setting of renal impairment. However, CT scanning with oral contrast offers a more accurate modality to assess the stage and progress of the underlying cancer, and can also reveal bowel obstruction and the site of urinary tract obstruction. In this particular patient the CT confirmed disease progression in the retroperitoneum and pelvis with external compression of the ureters, resulting in bilateral hydronephrosis. Magnetic resonance imaging (MRI) is not routinely indicated, but can be helpful if abnormal renal function precludes performing contrast-enhanced CT.

Patient management

The management of patients with malignant urinary tract obstruction poses a significant challenge and should be guided by symptom management and prognosis. Primary tumour site, performance status, tumour stage, therapeutic options and the patient's wishes are the main determining factors. Patients with newly diagnosed malignancies require multidisciplinary input to conserve renal function during the diagnostic work-up and histological confirmation. Some of these patients will have curable cancers or achieve significant benefit from palliative interventions.

Patients with complete bilateral obstruction and electrolyte abnormalities, including hyperkalaemia, require emergency intervention under the guidance of acute physicians supported by oncological advice. Haemodialysis is rarely indicated in patients with malignant obstructive uropathy, particularly those with end -stage disease.[5]

Lower urinary tract obstruction, including bladder outlet obstruction, should be managed with urgent urinary catheterization and consultation with the urological services. Further management will depend on the underlying malignancy, prior therapy and the patient's fitness for active medical or surgical treatment. Patients with advanced hormone-resistant prostate cancer have a high mortality rate during hospitalization and are unlikely to benefit from percutaneous nephrostomy (PCN).[5–7]

Upper urinary tract obstruction requires percutaneous decompression with nephrostomy. Although PCN is a safe and effective procedure and can result in rapid correction of biochemical parameters, it may be complicated by sepsis, obstruction and catheter loss. Typically, decompression is a two-stage process in the acute setting, involving a unilateral procedure followed by a decision on ureteric stenting at a later time. It should be noted that the relief of urosepsis is an acute emergency treated with nephrostomy and may give rapid improvement.

Conclusion

Patients with terminal-stage cancer and poor performance status, particularly those who have exhausted standard treatment options, may be best placed to receive supportive palliative care unless PCN or stenting is done in order to relief distressing symptoms or sepsis. These decisions require close collaboration with the acute oncology team, palliative care services and site-specific teams, while also taking into consideration the wishes of both the patient and their family. In a small retrospective case series, the median survival following PCN insertion was only 87 days. A majority of patients (79%) were able to be discharged from hospital. However, patients were re-admitted to hospital on average 1.6 times prior to their death through PCN-related or internal ureteric stent-related events.[8] Thus, in some patients, relief of obstruction by an invasive procedure may result in unnecessary pain and suffering without a clear quality of life gain.[8,9] Strict selection criteria should be applied to patients with a history of abdominopelvic malignancy before proceeding to PCN. No worthwhile benefit is obtained if nephrostomy is used as a palliative measure in the absence of definitive treatment.

Further Reading

1   Lau KO, Hia TN, Cheng C, Tay SK. Outcome of obstructive uropathy after pelvic irradiation in patients with carcinoma of the uterine cervix. *Ann Acad Med Singapore* 1998; **27**(5): 631-5.

2   Wong LM, Cleeve LK, Milner AD, Pitman AG. Malignant ureteral obstruction: outcomes after intervention. Have things changed? *J Urol* 2007; **178**: 178–83.

3   Yeung SJ, Escalante CP, editors. *Holland–Frei Oncologic Emergencies.* Hamilton, ON: BC Decker Inc; 2002.

4   Lienert A, Ing A, Mark S. Prognostic factors in malignant ureteric obstruction. *BJU* 2009; **104** (7): 938-41

5   Frederico RR, Broglio M, Silvio R, *et al.* Indications for percutaneous nephrostomy in patients with obstructive uropathy due to malignant urogenital neoplasia. *Int Braz J Urol* 2005; **31**(2): 117–24.

6   Chitale SV, Scott-Barrett S, Ho ET, Burgess NA. The management of ureteric obstruction secondary to malignant pelvic disease. *Clin Radiol* 2002; **57**: 1118–21.

7   Chiou RK, Chang WY, Horan JJ. Ureteral obstruction associated with prostate cancer: the outcome after percutaneous nephrostomy. *J Urol* 1990; **143**: 957–9.

8   Wilson JR, Urwin GH, Stower MJ. The role of percutaneous nephrostomy in malignant ureteric obstruction. *Ann R Coll Surg Engl* 2005; **87**: 21–4.

9   Watkinson AF, A'Hern RP, Jones A, King DM, Moskovic EC. The role of percutaneous nephrostomy in malignant urinary tract obstruction. *Clin Radiol* 1993; **47**(1): 32–5.

37 Management of Malignant Ascites in the Acute Oncology Setting

Anoop Haridass, Neil Kapoor, Helen Neville-Webbe

Case history

A 66-year-old woman with known advanced ovarian cancer has repeated emergency admission to her local district general hospital with symptomatic large-volume ascites. On each occasion, the patient is assessed in the emergency unit and subsequently admitted to a general medical ward for percutaneous drainage and symptomatic relief. The patient presents once again despite the recent completion of third-line chemotherapy.

What is ascites and what is the differential diagnosis?

What investigations would you perform?

What are the treatment options?

How would you manage this patient?

Background

What is ascites and what is the differential diagnosis?

Ascites is the accumulation of fluid within the peritoneal cavity, with the commonest cause being secondary to benign liver cirrhosis and portal hypertension. Approximately 10% of ascites cases are due to malignancy,[1] most commonly from primary ovarian, colon, stomach, pancreas, lung and breast cancers, but it can also be associated with primary liver or peritoneal mesothelial cancers. Ascites can be caused by occlusion of the draining lymphatic channels by malignant cells, massive liver metastases causing portal hypertension, or primary liver cancer in the setting of cirrhosis. Mean survival once malignant ascites is diagnosed is approximately one to four months.

Differential diagnosis

For patients presenting acutely with ascites, a high index of suspicion for an underlying process of malignancy should be countenanced. Benign causes should be excluded, including ascites secondary to liver cirrhosis (approximately 80% of cases), congestive cardiac failure, portal hypertension and chronic pancreatitis.

What investigations would you perform?

The aim of initial investigation is to diagnose the underlying condition causing ascites, whether benign or malignant; and, in the acute oncology setting, to also direct investigations which will lead to diagnosing the primary malignancy. Studies have shown that a serum-ascites albumin gradient (SAAG) of >1.1 g/dl is a useful test because it can identify patients with benign portal hypertension who will benefit from diuretic therapy (Figure 37.1).[2] The SAAG only needs to be determined at the first presentation with albumin measurements in the serum and ascitic fluid. Blood tests for complete blood count, liver function tests, and urea and electrolytes are helpful to exclude anaemia, infection, hypoalbuminaemia, liver dysfunction and renal dysfunction. If infection is suspected, ascitic fluid can be analysed for cell counts and culture of microorganisms. On first presentation, cytology of ascitic fluid can be performed, but tissue diagnosis following biopsy of solid tumour is more helpful in establishing the diagnosis. Therefore, on initial presentation, a computed tomography (CT) scan is required to further identify the disease process, and, in the case of malignancy, aid identification of a primary tumour and stage disease. If paracentesis is planned, a coagulation profile is also recommended. Tumour markers, such as CA125 (MUC16) and carcinoembryonic antigen (CEA), have poor

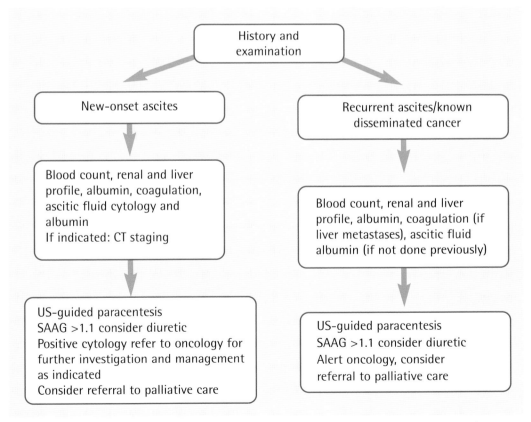

Figure 37.1 Management of suspected malignant ascites. CT, computed tomography; SAAG, serum-ascites albumin gradient; US, ultrasound.

sensitivity and specificity and their use in the diagnostic pathway for new-onset ascites should be discouraged.[3] However, should an ovarian or bowel mass be identified on scanning it is then entirely appropriate to employ relevant tumour markers.

What are the treatment options?

The aim of treatment is to alleviate the physical symptoms of ascites as soon as possible and enable speedy discharge from hospital, especially for patients in whom the malignant diagnosis is known and who require repeat admission to hospital due to ascites accumulation.

Paracentesis

This is the mainstay of managing malignant ascites. Paracentesis of up to 5 l of ascites can be safely carried out with minimal risk of hypotension and renal failure.[4] This provides quick (albeit temporary) relief of symptoms, such as distension, dyspnoea, nausea, early satiety and constipation. Larger-volume paracentesis may require clamping after every 4–5 l to allow time for the haemodynamic system to adjust. It is important to emphasize that, unlike with benign ascites, intravenous fluid replacement is largely not required to prevent hypotension in patients undergoing paracentesis for malignant ascites (who do not also have portal hypertension). However, bacterial peritonitis, loculation of the ascites, adhesions, and inadvertent puncturing of an organ with the ascitic needle are among the risks of paracentesis, albeit with a low incidence.

Diuretics

Diuretics are very commonly used but are only useful in 50% of cases.[5] If the patient has a SAAG of >1.1 g/dl use of a diuretic that affects the reninangiotensin axis is recommended (e.g. spironolactone 25–100 mg).

Other treatments

Peritoneo-venous shunt has been used effectively in cancer patients with a longer prognosis, but this needs a specialist surgical team and has significant side effects, such as pulmonary embolism, coagulation disorders, infection and shunt blockage.

Recent Developments

Peritoneal catheter

The PleurX peritoneal catheter and drainage system has recently been approved by the National Institute for Health and Care Excellence (NICE) for use in patients with recurrent malignant ascites.[6] This device consists of a silicone peritoneal catheter that is permanently placed inside the abdominal cavity with a cuff that is placed subcutaneously, and a safety valve on the abdominal wall of the patient. A vacuum bottle can be intermittently attached to the port to enable drainage of ascitic fluid by the patient or their community carer, so reducing the need for hospitalization. When not in use the valve is covered with a cap and a simple dressing. The advantage is that hospital admissions and repeat admissions are avoided, which is important for patients' quality of life, in addition to being cost-effective.

Systemic therapy of underlying malignancy

Treatment of the underlying malignancy with chemotherapy/surgery and biological agents can be helpful in controlling the ascites – especially in ovarian and breast cancer – and should be considered in patients who are fit enough for this approach. Intraperitoneal chemotherapy and antiangiogenic agents have also been used in a trial setting for ovarian cancer. Peritoneal dissemination of primary gastrointestinal cancer (stomach and pancreas) or lung cancer are associated with very poor prognosis, and patients are usually not fit enough to undergo treatment of the primary cancer.

How would you manage this patient?

In the case cited above, the patient was referred to the acute oncology team, which recommended insertion of a PleurX peritoneal catheter and drainage system. This was done within the radiology department on the day of admission. Following instruction in its use by the acute oncology nurse specialist, the patient was discharged home later that day, with community follow-up by the district nurse and her oncology consultant. The patient did not require further hospital admission for ascites.

Conclusions

The presence of ascites represents a symptom of serious underlying pathology. The aim of management is to establish the underlying cause in addition to providing rapid relief of symptoms by urgent drainage of ascites. For patients presenting with recurrent malignant ascites, rapid relief is essential to their physical and mental wellbeing, since prevention is not possible. Drainage should occur on the day of admission (preferably under ultrasound-guided control), and for those patients in whom the underlying disease is considered resistant to systemic treatment insertion of a PleurX peritoneal catheter enables admission avoidance and self-management within the community.

Further Reading

1 Beckera G, Galandib D, Bluma HE, *et al*. Malignant ascites: systematic review and guideline for treatment. *Eur J Cancer* 2006; **42**: 589–97.

2 Runyon BA, Montano AA, Akriviadis EA, *et al*. The serum-ascites albumin gradient is superior to the exudate-transudate concept in the differential diagnosis of ascites. *Ann Intern Med* 1992; **117**(3): 215–20.

3 Chen SJ, Wang SS, Lu CW, *et al*. Clinical value of tumour markers and serum-ascites albumin gradient in the diagnosis of malignancy-related ascites. *J Gastroenterol Hepatol* 1994; **9**(4): 396–400.

4 McNamara P. Paracentesis – an effective method of symptom control in the palliative care setting? *Palliat Med* 2000; **14**: 62–4.

5 Lee CW, Bociek G, Faught W. A survey of practices in management of malignant ascites. *J Pain Symptom Manage* 1998; **16**: 96–100.

6 National Institute for Health and Clinical Excellence [Internet]. *The PleurX peritoneal catheter drainage system for vacuum-assisted drainage of treatment-resistant, recurrent malignant ascites (MTG9)*. London: National Institute for Health and Care Excellence. c.2013. [Issued Mar 2012]. Available from: http://guidance.nice.org.uk/MTG9

38 Malignant Pleural Effusion

Judith Carser, Martin Ledson

Case history

A 70-year-old woman presented to her general physician (GP) with increasing shortness of breath on exertion over a two-month period. The patient's symptoms had deteriorated significantly within the last week and she was admitted as an emergency to her local emergency department. On admission, her performance status was 2 on the Eastern Cooperative Oncology Group (ECOG) score. The patient had a past medical history of a mastectomy and axillary node clearance for a T3 N0, ER-positive infiltrating ductal carcinoma of the left breast eight years ago, and received adjuvant radiotherapy and tamoxifen but had declined chemotherapy.

What is the differential diagnosis?

What are the appropriate investigations?

How would you manage this patient?

Background

What is the differential diagnosis?

There are many causes of shortness of breath in patients with a current or past history of cancer. In this case, the acute presentation against a background of chronic symptoms may have been triggered by a thromboembolic or cardiac event, or infection. In a patient with a prior history of cancer, malignant disease (including pleural or pericardial effusions), lymphangitis carcinomatosis, and disease progression due to pulmonary metastases should be considered.

What are the appropriate investigations?

An accurate history of the duration and onset of shortness of breath, including whether acute or chronic, together with associated symptoms such as fever, cough, chest pain or haemoptysis is important in determining the likely diagnosis, as is establishing if there is any history of prior lung disease or smoking. In this case, it was very important to elicit the past history of malignancy, since this adds a number of further differentials to the diagnostic list as breast cancer may relapse after a long disease-free interval.

A full history and clinical examination, including vital signs, should be performed. Typically a fluid collection of 500 ml can be detected clinically, with reduced air entry on the affected side and dullness to percussion. Blood tests that include biochemistry, haematology and inflammatory markers may be useful if infection is suspected. Initial radiological investigations should include a chest X-ray. This patient's chest X-ray (Figure 38.1) demonstrates a left pleural effusion together with loss of the left breast shadow. Pleural aspiration under ultrasound guidance confirmed a diagnosis of recurrent metastatic breast cancer on cytology. Samples should also be sent for protein, lactate dehydrogenase (LDH) and Gram stain if a diagnosis has not already been established to allow assessment of whether the effusion is an exudate or transudate.[1] Full staging with a computed tomography (CT) scan of chest and abdomen is indicated for patients in whom anticancer therapy is planned (Figure 38.2).

Typically, breast cancer is the most common presentation of a malignant pleural effusion in women, with lung cancer the most common cause in men, together accounting for over 50%–65% of all malignant effusions.[2] It is important to remember that not all pleural effusions in patients with cancer are necessarily malignant and may instead be associated with heart failure, pulmonary embolus or infection.

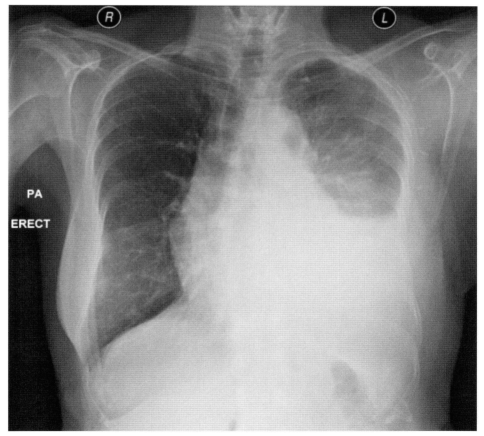

Figure 38.1 Chest X-ray demonstrates moderate–large left pleural effusion together with loss of the left breast shadow.

How would you manage this patient?

Treatment depends on a number of factor, which include the patient's symptoms at presentation, performance status, histology, burden of disease and chance of response to systemic therapy. If this is the first presentation, then a diagnosis must first be established with referral to the appropriate site-specific team. If the patient is presenting with relapsed disease from a previous cancer then liaison with the primary oncologist is appropriate.

The presence of malignant cells within the pleural cavity is usually associated with a poor prognosis, with median survival times 3–12 months.[3] Patients with breast and ovarian malignancies tend to have a better prognosis than those with lung or unknown primary cancers, due to the responsiveness of the underlying disease to systemic anticancer therapy.

Management options include surveillance, therapeutic aspiration, medical or surgical thoracoscopy and pleurodesis, or an indwelling pleural catheter (Figure 38.3).

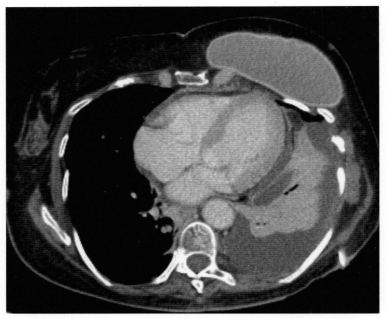

Figure 38.2 CT scan demonstrating left pleural effusion with associated collapse. Left breast prosthesis also noted.

Surveillance may be appropriate if the patient is asymptomatic and/or commencing systemic therapy for a responsive cancer. Many patients, however, will be symptomatic and require intervention. Therapeutic aspiration is not recommended for patients with a life expectancy of less than one month since the risk of re-accumulation requiring further intervention is high. Repeated aspiration can result in the formation of adhesions, which may make insertion of chest drains or thoracoscopic procedures more difficult. For frail patients, however, where the prognosis is poor, aspiration may be adequate to provide immediate symptom relief and avoid hospital admission. Current guidelines recommend that no more than 1.5l of fluid is removed at any one time because there is a risk of rebound pulmonary oedema.[2]

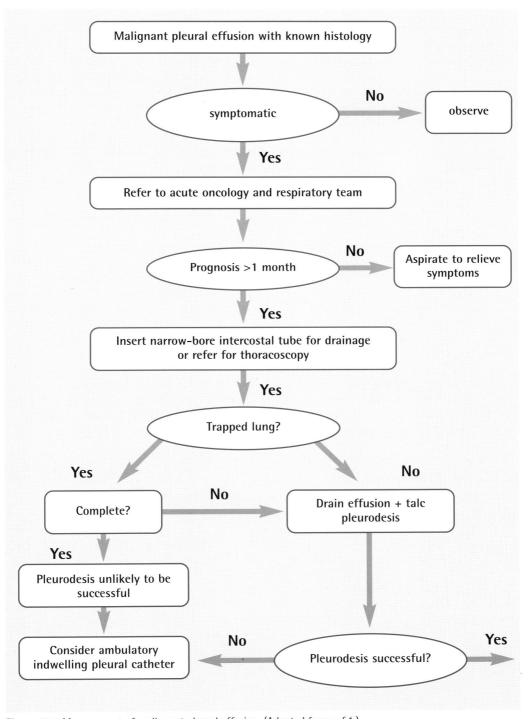

Figure 38.3 Management of malignant pleural effusion. (Adapted from ref.1.).

For all other patients, referral to a respiratory physician for consideration of a small-bore chest drain (10–14 Fr) and intrapleural instillation of a chemical sclerosant is recommended. Talc pleurodesis is the preferred option, with success rates of 80%–90%.[2,4] Chest drain insertion should be performed under ultrasound guidance since this increases the accuracy of the procedure and reduces the risk of iatrogenic organ damage.[1] Either medical or surgical thoracoscopy (video-assisted) and talc pleurodesis is the treatment of choice for good performance status patients, with success rates of 77%–100%. Video-assisted thoracic surgery (VATS) is particularly useful if both diagnosis and drainage of pleural fluid is required, as this can be done during one procedure. Video-assisted thoracic surgery is the most invasive method and requires a general anaesthetic, but VATS may also be indicated if lysis of intrapleural adhesions or partial decortication is required for trapped lung (failure of lung to re-expand following drainage). Currently there is no direct comparative evidence to suggest whether surgical or medical pleurodesis is superior, and the choice may depend on local service arrangements.[5]

Ambulatory indwelling pleural catheters may be useful in controlling symptoms in patients with recurrent malignant effusions after failure of talc pleurodesis, though spontaneous pleurodesis occurs in some patients. This can be a useful option to reduce repeated hospital admissions, especially for patients towards the end of life, although adverse events such as catheter blockage and infection are more common than with talc pleurodesis.[6] Intrapleural instillation of fibrinolytic agents such as streptokinase or urokinase may be useful in patients with resistant multiloculated effusions.[7]

Systemic anticancer therapy may be useful in controlling symptoms from pleural effusions in chemosensitive malignancies small such as cell lung cancer, breast cancer, ovarian cancer and lymphoma. In many cases, however, other therapeutic interventions are required. Tumour seeding is uncommon following pleural procedures, and, other than for patients with a diagnosis of malignant pleural mesothelioma, prophylactic port site radiotherapy is not recommended.[2]

Conclusion

Acute presentations with symptoms secondary to a malignant pleural effusion require a multidisciplinary team approach with assessment by the acute oncology, respiratory and thoracic surgery teams to determine appropriate management. This will primarily be determined by the patient's performance status and symptoms, but must also take into account the nature and burden of disease, likelihood of response to systemic therapy (including prognosis), and whether this is a new or recurrent presentation. Close links with palliative care and community nursing services are crucial, and interventions should be aimed at maximizing symptom control while reducing the need for hospital attendances. The potential for elective day case pleural aspiration should be explored as a means of maximizing patient experience and reducing hospital admissions.

Further reading

1 Hooper C, Lee YC, Maskell N. Investigation of a unilateral pleural effusion in adults: British Thoracic Society Pleural Disease Guideline 2010. *Thorax* 2010; **65**(Suppl 2): ii4–ii17.

2 Roberts, ME, Neville E, Berrisford RG, Antunes G, Ali NJ; BTS Pleural Disease Guideline Group. Management of a malignant pleural effusion: British Thoracic Society Pleural Disease Guideline 2010. *Thorax* 2010; **65**(Suppl 2): ii32–ii40.

3 Burrows CM, Mathews WC, Colt HG. Predicting survival in patients with recurrent symptomatic malignant pleural effusions: an assessment of the prognostic values of physiologic, morphologic, and quality of life measures of extent of disease. *Chest* 2000; **117**(1): 73–8.

4 Shaw P, Agarwal R. Pleurodesis for malignant pleural effusions. *Cochrane Database Syst Rev* 2004; **1**: CD002916.

5 Dresler CM, Olak J, Herndon JE 2nd, *et al.* Phase III intergroup study of talc poudrage vs talc slurry sclerosis for malignant pleural effusion. *Chest* 2005; **127**(3): 909–15.

6 Davies HE, Mishra EK, Kahan BC, *et al.* Effect of an indwelling pleural catheter vs chest tube and talc pleurodesis for relieving dyspnea in patients with malignant pleural effusion: the TIME2 randomized controlled trial. *JAMA* 2012; **307**(22): 2383–9.

7 Davies CW, Traill ZC, Gleeson FV, Davies RJ. Intrapleural streptokinase in the management of malignant multiloculated pleural effusions. *Chest* 1999; **115**(3): 729–33.

39 Metabolic Complications of Malignancy: Hypercalcaemia

Eliyaz Ahmed, Richard Griffiths, Sid McNulty

Case history

A 73-year-old man with a renal cell carcinoma and pulmonary metastases has been under surveillance for three years. He is referred to the surgical assessment unit with a three-day history of abdominal pains associated with constipation, nausea and profound fatigue. On examination the patient appears dry with loss of skin turgor, and he appears to be disorientated in time and place. His biochemistry reveals a urea of 24 mmol/l, creatinine 363 mmol/l and a corrected calcium of 3.4 mmol/l.

What are the causes of hypercalcaemia?

What is the differential diagnosis?

How would you manage this patient?

Background

What are the causes of hypercalcaemia?

Around 30% of patients with known malignancy will develop hypercalcaemia at some stage of the disease.[1] Breast, lung and renal carcinomas, multiple myeloma and lymphomas are the most common malignancies associated with hypercalcaemia. Patients usually have disseminated disease and this portends a poor prognosis with a median survival of 3–4 months.

The pathophysiology of hypercalcaemia in malignancy involves an interplay of factors that disrupt the normal calcium homeostasis. In many cases, hypercalcaemia may be a consequence of both humoral and tumour-directed osteolytic effects on the bone. In humoral hypercalcaemia of malignancy, the hypercalcaemia is mediated by the tumor secreting parathyroid hormone-related protein (PTHrP), which mimics the actions of parathyroid hormone on calcium metabolism. Other mechanisms include overproduction of vitamin D, as seen in haematological cancers such as lymphoma.[2] It is important to remember that patients can develop hypercalcaemia without bone involvement.[3]

What is the differential diagnosis?

Clinical manifestations are non-specific with a variety of systemic symptoms (Table 39.1) and hypercalcaemia is often discovered on a routine blood screen. As circulating calcium is bound to albumin the total serum calcium levels can be affected by changes in plasma albumin; therefore, calcium levels need to be corrected for albumin levels.

Hypercalcaemia may be secondary to primary hyperparathyroidism, hence, calcium and PTH should be measured at baseline. A normal or raised PTH in the presence of a raised calcium is abnormal and suggests hyperparathyroidism (primary or tertiary) as the cause of the raised calcium. If PTH is suppressed then it suggests another cause, such as PTHrP.[4] Other differential diagnoses include thiazide diuretics, granulomatous diseases and lymphoma.

Table 39.1 Clinical features of hypercalcaemia	
Neurological	**Gastrointestinal**
Impaired concentration	Nausea and vomiting
Confusion	Anorexia
Apathy	Abdominal pain
Headaches	Constipation
Drowsiness/obtundation	**Cardiovascular**
Lethargy	
Muscle weakness	Hypertension
	Bradycardia
Renal	Prolonged PR interval, widened QRS, shortened
Polyuria	QT interval
Polydipsia	Bundle branch/ atrioventricular blocks
Nocturia	
Renal stones	
Renal failure	

How would you manage this patient?

Withdraw thiazide diuretics and sources of vitamin A and vitamin D. The majority of patients with significant hypercalcaemia have intravascular volume depletion, and vigorous rehydration and expansion of intravascular volume that promotes calcium excretion is the mainstay of treatment. Careful monitoring for signs of overload and electrolytes is required.

Bisphosphonates are the most effective agents to reduce calcium levels – these work by inhibiting osteoclastic bone resorption. Pamidronic acid or zoledronic acid are commonly used, though zoledronic acid has shown to be more efficacious in reducing calcium levels.[5] Dialysis is an option when renal or cardiac failure precludes the use of vigorous hydration or use of bisphosphonates. Mithramycin (plicamycin) and gallium nitrate are rarely used at present, but considered when bisphosphonates are ineffective.

Calcitonin (intramuscular or subcutaneous at a dose of 4–8 IU/kg every 12 hours) is useful when urgent reduction of calcium levels is required, particularly in patients with seizures and arrhythmias. Development of tachyphylaxis is a problem and therefore it is not used alone.

Corticosteroids are mainly used for treatment of hypercalcaemia associated with haematological malignancies such as lymphoma.

Treatment of the underlying malignancy is an important aspect of care in all cases of malignancy-associated hypercalcaemia.

Recent Developments

Receptor activator of nuclear factor κB (RANK) is a transmembrane signalling receptor expressed on osteoclast precursor cells and its ligand, the RANK ligand (RANKL), is a key mediator of osteoclast-induced bone resorption. Denosumab, a monoclonal antibody that binds RANKL, has been approved for prevention of skeletal-related events in bone secondaries from solid tumors.[6] Randomized control trials have not only shown superior efficacy of denosumab over zoledronic acid, but treatment with denosumab is associated with a decreased incidence or delayed onset of malignancy-associated hypercalcaemia.[7,8] Denosumab has the potential for use in the treatment of malignancy-associated hypercalcaemia, given the reported effects of hypocalcaemia and decreased incidence of hypercalcaemia associated with denosumab as reported in clinical trials. Furthermore, published case reports add credence to its potential in the management of malignancy-associated hypercalcaemia.[9] A randomized clinical trial is under way to address the efficacy of denosumab in the treatment of hypercalcaemia of malignancy refractory to bisphosphonates.[10]

Conclusions

Hypercalcaemia is a common complication of malignancy and patients usually have widespread disease at presentation. A combination of vigorous saline hydration and antiresorptive agents is the mainstay of treatment, along with treatment of the underlying malignancy. Inhibitors of RANKL, which are efficacious in preventing skeletal-related events, may also prove useful in the management of hypercalcaemia.

Further Reading

1   Vassilopoulou-Sellin R, Newman BM, Taylor SH, Guinee VF. Incidence of hypercalcemia in patients with malignancy referred to a comprehensive cancer center. *Cancer* 1993; **71**: 1309–12.

2   Stewart AF. Clinical practice. Hypercalcemia associated with cancer. *N Engl J Med* 2005; **352**: 373–9.

3   Grill V, Martin TJ. Hypercalcemia of malignancy. *Rev Endocr Metab Disord* 2000; **1**: 253–63.

4   Hutchesson AC, Bundred NJ, Ratcliffe WA. Survival in hypercalcaemic patients with cancer and co-existing primary hyperparathyroidism. *Postgrad Med J* 1995; **71**(831): 28–31.

5   Major P, Lortholary A, Hon J, *et al.* Zoledronic acid is superior to pamidronate in the treatment of hypercalcemia of malignancy: a pooled analysis of two randomized, controlled clinical trials. *J Clin Oncol* 2001; **19**: 558–67.

6   Baron R, Ferrari S, Russell RG. Denosumab and bisphosphonates: Different mechanisms of action and effects. *Bone* 2011; **48**: 677–92.

7   Lipton A, Stopeck A, Von Moos R. A meta-analysis of results from two randomized, double blind studies of denosumab versus zoledronic acid for treatment of bone metastases. *J Clin Oncol* 2010; **28**: A9015.

8   Diel IJ, Body JJ, Stopeck A, *et al.* Effect of denosumab treatment on prevention of
    hypercalcemia of malignancy in cancer patients with bone metastasis. Abstract number 3051.
    Presented at the European Multidisciplinary Cancer Congress; 23–27 Sep 2011; Stockholm,
    Sweden.

9   Boikos SA, Hammers H. Denosumab for the treatment of bisphosphonate-refractory
    hypercalcemia. *J Clin Oncol* 2012; **30**(29): e299.

10 Hu MI, Gucalp R, Insogna KL, *et al.* Single-arm multicenter proof-of-concept study of
    denosumab to treat hypercalcemia of malignancy in patients who are refractory to IV
    bisphosphonates. *J Clin Oncol* 2011; **29**(suppl): Abstract TPS245.

40 Metabolic Complications of Malignancy: Hyponatraemia

Eliyaz Ahmed, Richard Griffiths, Sid McNulty

Case history

A 62-year-old female smoker with chronic obstructive airways disease presents to the emergency department with a collapse. She gives a six-week history of cough, anorexia and weight loss with recent onset of dizziness, nausea and confusion. The admitting doctor noted that she was vague, with an abbreviated mental test score of 7 out of 10. A chest X-ray shows a large mass at the right hilum with widening of the mediastinum. Her serum sodium returns at 111 mmol/l.

What is the differential diagnosis?

How would you manage this patient?

Background

Hyponatraemia occurs when there is an excess of water in the extracellular fluid compartment relative to its sodium content. Patients can be asymptomatic, or they may report headache, difficulty concentrating, weakness, muscle cramps and dysgeusia. A rapid drop in sodium can cause more dramatic neurological manifestations, including confusion, seizures, reduced level of consciousness and respiratory arrest.

Hyponatraemia is commonly a consequence of excess sodium loss from either the gastrointestinal tract or the kidneys, or excess dilution due to cardiac, liver or renal impairment. In addition, patients with malignant disease, inappropriate diuresis is typically due to ectopic production of antidiuretic hormone by the tumour.[1-3] The patient should always be assessed in terms of their fluid volume status: are they hypo-, hyper- or euvolaemic? A careful drug history should always be sought, and other causes of hyponatraemia should be looked for before a diagnosis of syndrome of inappropriate antidiuretic hormone (SIADH) is made. Treatment of hyponatraemia involves correcting the underlying cause (Table 40.1), and, therefore, recognizing the pathophysiological process leading to low sodium is crucial in determining the most appropriate management.

What is the differential diagnosis?

Initially, the key differential is whether the hyponatraemia is caused by SIADH, fluid overload or depletion. A full history and physical examination should be undertaken, bearing in mind the differential diagnoses in Table 40.1. The key to understanding SIADH is the inappropriate levels of serum versus urine osmolality. If the serum is concentrated then the urine should be concentrated, and it would be inappropriate to have a dilute urine (which may be in the 'normal' range). Similarly, if the serum is dilute then the urine should be dilute, and it would be inappropriate to have a concentrated urine (which may be in the 'normal' range). The presence of SIADH is revealed by a dilute serum with an inappropriately concentrated urine. A paired urine and plasma osmolality can assist in the differential diagnosis: patients with SIADH typically appear euvolaemic and have concentrated urine relative to the plasma. Urinary osmolality in SIADH should be >100 mOsm with a plasma osmolality <275 mOsm (any value up to the serum level, i.e. 275 mOsm, is inappropriate when the samples are paired). A urinary sodium level >40 mmol/l is also helpful in confirming the diagnosis. A urinary sodium of <30 mmol/l indicates that there may be contraction of the extracellular fluid compartment and infusion of 0.9% saline is indicated.[2,3]

How would you manage this patient?

Treatment of the underlying cause is the mainstay of treatment for hyponatraemia. However, patients with a sodium level <125 mmol/l normally would warrant further action to improve symptoms and reduce the likelihood of neurological deterioration. Fluid restriction is the mainstay of management of these patients while encouraging adequate protein and salt in the diet. To calculate the required amount of fluid restriction use the formula:

$$\frac{\text{Urinary Na} + \text{Urinary K}}{\text{Plasma Na}}$$

For values:	Restrict fluid to:
<1	1000 ml a day
~1	500–700 ml a day
>1	500 ml a day

Demeclocycline can also be effective in a dose of 300–600 mg twice daily, but can cause troublesome side effects including nausea. Demeclocycline can be nephrotoxic and patients should be warned of the potential for a photosensitive skin rash. The aim is to correct sodium levels by about 8 mmol/l per 24-hour period. A more rapid rise in sodium can precipitate osmotic demyelination in the brain stem, which is characterized by affective changes, dysarthria, quadriparesis and pseudobulbar palsy.

For patients who present acutely with seizures or coma urgent and careful correction of the plasma sodium is warranted, and in this situation 3% saline can be infused ensuring that the sodium does not rise by more than 1–2 mmol/l per hour and no more than 10 mmol/l in the first 24 hours. Some authors suggest the use of furosemide 20 mg intravenously if there are also signs of extracellular fluid overload (e.g. oedema).[2,4]

Table 40.1 Causes of hyponatraemia in cancer patients

Due to SIAD	**Intracranial pathology***
Malignancies	Infections – encephalitis and meningitis
Carcinoma of the lung (typically small-cell carcinoma)	Intracranial hemorrhage
Upper gastrointestinal carcinomas	Cerebral infarction
Transitional cell carcinomas of the urothelium	**Associated with increased extracellular fluid**
Ewing's sarcoma	Ascites
Lymphomas	Cirrhosis
Intracranial tumours	Congestive cardiac failure
	Nephrotic syndrome
Drugs	Renal failure
Selective serotonin reuptake inhibitors	
Carbamazepine	**Associated with reduced extracellular fluid**
Tricyclic antidepressants	Thiazide diuretics
Phenothiazines	Adrenal insufficiency
Opioids	Diarrhoea
Non-steroidal anti-inflammatory drugs	Vomiting
Post anaesthesia	
Cytotoxic drugs	
Cisplatin	
Vincristine	
Ifosfamide	
Cyclophosphamide	

*Can cause hyponatraemia through SIAD or by renal sodium loss, known as cerebral salt wasting. SIAD, syndrome of inappropriate antidiuretic hormone.

Fluid restriction, followed by consideration of demeclocycline, remains the first-line management for SIADH. However, vasopressin receptor antagonists have recently been introduced into clinical practice, which act by blocking the effect of vasopressin on its receptors in the renal collecting duct, thereby increasing clearance of free water. Tolvaptan is licensed in Europe for the correction of hyponatraemia secondary to SIADH, and has been shown to be significantly better than placebo at increasing sodium levels in patients with SIADH, heart failure and cirrhosis. It is used at a dose of 15–60 mg daily and patients are encouraged to drink freely. Side effects include thirst, dry mouth and increased urine volume. Daily measurement of electrolytes is required on initiation. In studies, 1.8% of patients experienced too rapid a rise in sodium and 1.1% experienced overcorrection of sodium, although no neurological events were observed as a result of this. There are currently no good data on the effect this class of drug has on clinically relevant outcomes such as quality of life, morbidity and mortality.[5]

Conclusions

Hyponatraemia is the most common electrolyte abnormality in cancer patients, is frequently associated with an adverse prognosis, and can affect quality of life. A thorough history, examination and biochemical assessment can assist in determining the cause to allow the most effective management. Correction of hyponatraemia needs to be done carefully, with serial monitoring of electrolytes. The newer class of vasopressin receptor inhibitors may have a role to play, but more data is needed on how these drugs can affect clinically meaningful end points.

Further reading

1   Onitilo AA, Kio E, Doi, SA. Tumor-related hyponatremia. *Clin Med Res* 2007; **5**(4): 228–37.

2   Ellison DH, Berl T. The syndrome of inappropriate antidiuresis. *N Engl J Med* 2007; **356**: 2064–72.

3   Adrogue HJ, Madias NE. Hyponatremia. *N Engl J Med* 2000; **342**: 1581–9.

4   Verbalis JG, Goldsmith SR, Grennberg A, *et al.* Hyponatremia treatment guidelines: expert panel recommendations. *Am J Med* 2007; **120**(suppl1): S1–S21.

5   Verbalis JG, Adler S, Schrier RW, *et al.* Efficacy and safety of oral tolvaptan in patients with the syndrome of inappropriate antidiuretic hormone secretion. *Eur J Endocrinol* 2011; **164**(5): 725–32.

PROBLEM

41 Bowel Obstruction in Acute Oncology

Mike Scott, John Green

Case history

A 59-year-old woman presents with abdominal distension against a background of advanced ovarian cancer with primary debulking surgery and multiple lines of palliative chemotherapy. Computed tomography (CT) scanning showed minimal ascites but progressive peritoneal nodules, including an indeterminate mass in the uterovaginal pouch. The pain became progressively worse over the next few days and was associated with faeculent vomiting. A plain X-ray of the abdomen showed small bowel obstruction.

What are the causes of malignant bowel obstruction?

What are the principles of management in this patient?

Background

What are the causes of malignant bowel obstruction?

Obstruction of the gastrointestinal (GI) tract is a not uncommon presenting feature of primary and recurrent colorectal cancers, and advanced or recurrent gynaecological malignancies. It accounts for 10% of the presentations of acute oncology. A proportion of these tumours will have their primary presentations as subacute obstruction through general surgical, GI and (less frequently) gynaecological cancer teams. The obstruction may be from a single site, as is most commonly the case in colorectal cancer where intraluminal disease is the major factor, or from multiple sites as a result of widespread intra-abdominal carcinomatosis, which cause mechanical disturbances of motility as well as involvement of mesenteric plexuses.[1] In the case of recurrent cancer, a multidisciplinary team approach the surgical and non-surgical management of bowel obstruction is required.[2] Where a palliative approach is adopted, management of the psychosocial issues of the patients and their families is required.

Non-malignant causes of bowel obstruction should always be considered, particularly where previous surgery has been performed or radiation has been given to the abdomen or pelvis (Table 41.1).[3,4]

Diagnosis and initial management

Diagnosis is based on the patient's history, clinical assessment and an initially plain abdominal X-ray. Pelvic examination may be helpful if relapse from a gynaecological primary is suspected and this provides a simple assessment of the extent of metastatic disease. Computed tomography is often helpful in delineating the site and extent of disease, although water-soluble oral contrast may be required and small-volume peritoneal disease may not be demonstrated. Where the patient is located in a medical assessment

Table 41.1 Causes of bowel obstruction

Extrinsic lesions	Intrinsic lesions	Obstruction of normal bowel lumen
Adhesions	Congenital malformations	Intussusception
Hernia	Duplication, atresia, stenosis	Gallstones
Volvulus	Neoplasm	Faeces or meconium
	Inflammatory stricture	Bezoar
	Radiation enteritis	Traumatic intramural haematoma

unit, close liaison with surgical teams is essential, and in the case of recurrent disease the responsible oncologist should be informed.

Although imaging will usually identify the site of bowel obstruction, opioid therapy and electrolyte imbalance may complicate the clinical picture, as may dysmotility caused by concurrent medication. In the immunosuppressed patient secondary infection is common and neutropenic enterocolitis, as well as cytomegalovirus, should always be considered in the differential diagnosis.

From the point of view of patient management, adequate fluid replacement and analgesia are essential during the early assessment period, as dehydration and severe pain are frequently seen.

Prognostic factors

In the case of a primary presentation, the prognosis is largely dictated by the type of the underlying cancer. A primary presentation of an advanced bowel cancer may be associated with an improved prognosis compared with recurrent ovarian cancer. Presentations with obstruction may, of course, reflect additional local factors such as advanced disease, and this is associated with an adverse prognosis. In advanced or recurrent disease, prognostic factors are as summarized in Table 41.2.

Table 41.2 Prognostic factors in malignant bowel obstruction

Favourable	Unfavourable
Good performance status	Poor performance status
Treatment-free interval >6 months	Treatment-free interval <6 months
Chemosensitivity	Chemoresistance
No/small-volume ascites	Large-volume ascites
Single-site disease	Multiple-site disease
Albumin >25 g/L	Albumin <25 g/L

What are the principles of management in this patient?

Surgical management

Depending on the site of the obstruction, a number of surgical options are available including resection, bypass, formation of a stoma and GI stenting.[5] Surgical intervention should be considered when symptoms have not been relieved after 48 hours of conservative medical management.

In the case of colonic obstruction it has been suggested that stenting may offer an equivalent benefit to surgery.[6] It should be highlighted that the mortality from surgery in this group of patients is in the range of 12%–30%, and morbidity may be as high as 50%.

The overall palliation achieved by surgical intervention in patients with bowel obstruction has been estimated to be of the order of 60% at 60 days.[7]

Non-surgical management

1. General measures

Initial management is fasting, intravenous hydration with careful monitoring of electrolytes and albumin, and pain control. Enemas can be used if faecal impaction is thought to be contributory. A nasogastric tube may be inserted where vomiting is persistent, but should be regarded as a temporary measure while awaiting other treatment decisions. Good oral hygiene is essential. Total parenteral nutrition should be used with care and only for a defined period.[8,9] It is not recommended for most terminally ill patients and should be reserved for those with true long-term prognosis. Chemotherapy has not been shown to be beneficial in established cases of obstruction and may be detrimental in view of the association with an increased risk of infection and a small risk of GI perforation.[10]

2. Drug therapy

Steroids are widely used to reduce swelling in the bowel wall, although there is no category 1 evidence for their use. Dexamethasone at 4–16 mg subcutaneously daily may be helpful in treating incomplete small bowel obstruction, but should be discontinued after 4–5 days if not proving effective. Antiemetics may offer some symptomatic relief and often need to be given by continuous infusion. Pain control is important and should not be withheld, but the risk of opioid accumulation is considerable where renal decompensation is present. Motility agents such as metoclopramide may help in cases of incomplete obstruction, but are contraindicated in complete bowel obstruction. Antisecretory agents, e.g. octreotide, can relieve symptoms such as pain and nausea by reducing GI secretions.[11]

Conclusions

Bowel obstruction is a common presentation of primary GI tumours, but the onset is normally insidious. In advanced or recurrent disease of GI or ovarian origin, it is more commonly an acute presentation. The obstruction is more likely to be multifocal in gynaecological than in GI tumours. The presence of extensive disease or chemoresistance is associated with a poor prognosis and multidisciplinary discussion is required to ensure optimum management. Quality-of-life data are sparse. Clear national guidelines on this distressing complication of cancer are encouraged.

Further Reading

1   Ripamonti C, Bruera E. Palliative management of malignant bowel obstruction. *Int J Gynecol Cancer* 2002; **12**: 135–43.

2   Feuer DJ, Broadley KE, Shepherd JH, Barton DPJ. Systematic review of surgery in malignant bowel obstruction in advanced gynaecological and gastrointestinal cancer. *Gynecol Oncol* 1999; **75**: 313–22.

3   Jatoi A, Podratz KC, Gill P, Hartmann LC. Pathophysiology and palliation of inoperable bowel obstruction in patients with ovarian cancer. *J Support Oncol* 2004; **2**: 323–37.

4   Montz FJ, Holschneider CH, Solh S, *et al*. Small bowel obstruction following radical hysterectomy: risk factors, incidence and operative findings. *Gynecol Oncol* 1994; **53**: 114–20.

5   Jolicoeur L, Faught W. Managing bowel obstruction in ovarian cancer using a percutaneous endoscopic gastrostomy (PEG) tube. *Can Oncol Nurs J* 2003: **13**(4): 213–9.

6   Van Hooft J, Bemelman WA, Oldeburg B, *et al*. Colonic stenting versus emergency surgery for acute left-sided malignant colonic obstruction: a multicentre randomised trial. *Lancet Oncol* 2011; **12**: 344–52.

7   Kolomainen DF, Barton DPJ. Surgical management of bowel obstruction in gynaecological malignancies. *Curr Opin Support Palliat Care* 2011; **5**: 55–9.

8   Kucukmetin A, Naik R, Galaal K, Bryant A, Dickinson HO. Palliative surgery versus medical management for bowel obstruction in ovarian cancer. *Cochrane Database Syst Rev* 2010; **7**: CD007792.

9   Rousseau P. Management of malignant bowel obstruction in advanced cancer: a brief overview. *J Palliat Med* 1998; **1**(1): 65–72.

10 Perren TJ, Swart AM, Pfisterer J, *et al*. A phase 3 trial of bevacizumab in ovarian cancer. *N Engl J Med* 2011; **365**: 2484–96.

11 Mystakidou K, Tsilika E, Kalaidopoulou O, *et al*. Comparison of octreotide administration versus conservative treatment in the management of inoperable bowel obstruction in patients with advanced cancer: a randomised double blind controlled trial. *Anticancer Res* 2002; **22**: 1187–92.

42 Malignant Pericardial Effusion

Madhuchanda Chatterjee, Judith Carser, Nick Palmer

Case history

A 49-year-old woman, established on palliative endocrine therapy for metastatic breast cancer, was admitted to hospital with shortness of breath. She had a past medical history of breast surgery, adjuvant radiotherapy and adjuvant endocrine therapy with tamoxifen. Her disease progressed with nodal, mediastinal and pulmonary metastases after three years. She had documented bony metastases affecting the sternum. On admission she was noted to be hypotensive with a sinus tachycardia and hypoxia.

What is the differential diagnosis?

What are the appropriate investigations?

How would you manage this patient?

Background

What is the differential diagnosis?

Shortness of breath can be a common feature in patients with malignancy due to the primary tumour or metastases and may be due to:

- thromboembolic event
- drug-related cardiac failure
- infection
- development of pleural or pericardial effusion
- anaemia.

In this case, the patient was also haemodynamically compromised. Additional clinical signs suggesting pericardial effusion would be:

- raised jugular venous pressure
- if cardiac tamponade is evident pulsus paradoxus may be present (fall in inspiratory BP >10 mmHg)
- quiet or muffled heart sounds.

Common causes for large pericardial effusions are neoplasia, infection (e.g. tuberculosis), uraemia and myxoedema.[1] The finding of a pericardial effusion in a patient with known malignancy is commonly associated with metastatic spread.[2]

Patients with a history of thoracic radiotherapy can develop a radiation-induced pericarditis with a pericardial effusion. Development of infectious or autoimmune pericardial effusions is occasionally seen in immunocompromised patients due to treatment of their malignancy.

What are the appropriate investigations?

The presence of a pericardial effusion may be suspected in cancer patients with any condition affecting the pericardium, including acute pericarditis. Other clues are recurrent and persistent fever, unilateral pleural effusion associated with haemodynamic compromise, or cardiomegaly on the chest X-ray. Malignancy such as breast, lung or oesophageal cancer, metastatic melanoma, lymphoma and leukemia are the most common underlying diagnosis.[3-5] A full history of the duration of symptoms, along with past medical history and clinical examination (including vital signs assessing the haemodynamic impact) should be taken. Following this, an electrocardiogram (ECG), chest X-ray, and a full blood count with chemistry profile and renal function are required. Echocardiography is essential to establish the diagnosis of pericardial effusion, the haemodynamic impact of the effusion, and to check for concomitant heart disease or paracardial pathology. Cardiac tamponade, the decompensated phase of cardiac compression, develops when the intrapericardial pressure due to the increasing pericardial effusion is elevated enough to impair filling of the cardiac chambers, primarily the right ventricle. Tuberculosis, mediastinal irradiation and previous cardiac surgical procedures may lead to constrictive pericarditis with reduced preload and stroke volumes.

A pericardial effusion appears as an echolucent space between the pericardium and the epicardium. Effusions exceeding the physiologic amount of 25–50 ml are seen as an echo-free space during the whole cardiac cycle.

Characteristic ECG findings are low QRS voltage (QRS complexes ≤5 mm, 0.5 mV) in all limb leads and electrical alternans. In the ECG a 'swinging heart' is suggestive of pericardial effusion, cardiac tamponade or pericardial inflammation.

Chest X-ray is insensitive in detecting pericardial disease. A subacute cardiac tamponade may be suggested by an enlarged cardiac silhouette with clear lung fields (Figure 42.1).

Cardiac biomarkers, e.g. troponin and CK-MB, may be elevated in patients with acute pericarditis, and elevated leukocytes, lactate dehydrogenase (LDH) and erythrocyte sedimentation rate may indicate an infection.

Patients with a new diagnosis of pericardial effusion should be immediately referred to a cardiologist. Pericardiocentesis with cytology and pericardial biopsy should be performed to establish the underlying aetiology. Cytology with findings of malignant cells are more likely in haemorrhagic pericardial effusions than in non-haemorrhagic ones (Figure 42.2).[6]

How would you manage this patient?

The focus of treatment of a haemodynamically stable pericardial effusion is the underlying condition that is causing the effusion. The need for invasive therapeutic action is prompted by the presence of symptoms such as fatigue, dyspnoea or chest heaviness, and anticipated survival of the patient. Asymptomatic or least symptomatic pericardial effusion can be managed conservatively with repeated monitoring, avoidance of fluid

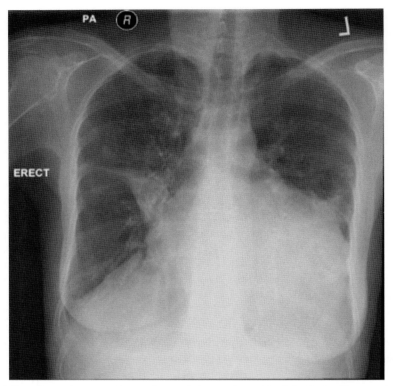

Figure 42.1 Chest X-ray demonstrating cardiomegaly in a patient with clinically significant pericardial effusion.

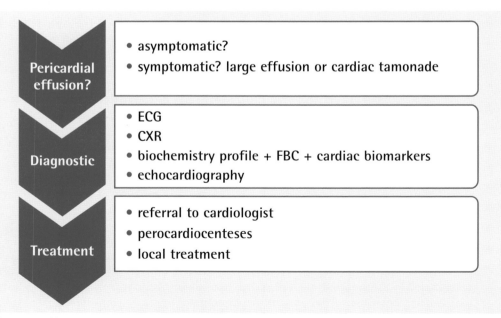

Figure 42.2 Management of pericardial effusion.

depletion and treatment of the underlying cause. Pericardial aspiration with culture and cytology of the aspirate may be useful to aid diagnosis, but should only be undertaken when there is a sufficient rim of fluid to approach.

Pericardiocentesis is life-saving in cardiac tamponade, and is performed under echocardiographic and X-ray guidance with an indwelling catheter placed in the pericardial space. In haemodynamically uncompromised patients a pericardiocentesis is indicated in effusions >20 mm on echocardiography in diastole, or used for diagnostic purposes to unveil the aetiology of the underlying cause (Figure 42.3).[7] A re-accumulation is seen in 60% of cases after pericardiocentesis.[8] Recurrence rates appear to be higher after simple pericardiocentesis or large-volume effusions.[7] Several measures can be attempted to prevent re-accumulation, including: prolonged catheter drainage;

Figure 42.3 Echocardiography of a malignant pericardial effusion pre- (A) and post-aspiration (B) of pericardial fluid demonstrating a reduction in the echolucent space.

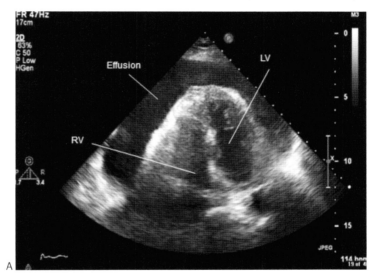

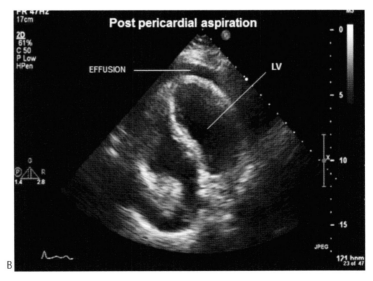

pericardial sclerosis with instillation of sclerosing agents such as tetracycline, doxycycline, minocycline, bleomycin and talc; and surgical decompression of the pericardium, known as pericardiotomy or pericardiectomy, using video-assisted thoracic surgery (VATS) and balloon pericardiotomy.

A symptomatic pericardial effusion in patients with a known malignancy is usually associated with a short life expectancy.[9] Intrapericardial chemotherapy (e.g. cisplatin) may be considered as a local treatment with minimum systemic side effects to reduce the recurrence rate of a haemodynamically compromising pericardial effusion.[10] In the case described above, the patient was transferred to the care of a cardiologist for an echocardiographic-guided pericardial drain, which relieved her symptoms.

Conclusion

The treatment of a pericardial effusion depends on the underlying condition. Therefore, multidisciplinary team working that involves acute oncology, surgical and cardiological assessment, and site-specific oncological assessment is necessary. The need for invasive treatment is prompted by the presence of symptoms and the anticipated survival of the patient.

Further reading

1   Merce J, Sagrista-Sauleda J, Permanyer-Miralda G, *et al.* Should pericardial drainage be performed routinely in patients who have a large pericardial effusion without tamponade? *Am J Med* 1998; **105**: 106–9.

2   Klatt EC, Heitz DR. Cardiac metastases. *Cancer* 1990; **65**: 1456–9.

3   Ben-Horin S, Bank I, Guetta V, Livneh A. Large symptomatic pericardial effusion as the presentation of unrecognized cancer: a study in 173 consecutive patients undergoing pericardiocentesis. *Medicine (Baltimore)* 2006; **85**: 49–53.

4   Gornik HL, Gerhard-Herman M, Beckman JA. Abnormal cytology predicts poor prognosis in cancer patients with pericardial effusion. *J Clin Oncol* 2005; **23**: 5211–6.

5   Sampat K, Rossi A, Garcia-Gutierrez V, *et al.* Characteristics of pericardial effusions in patients with leukemia. *Cancer* 2010; **116**: 2366–71.

6   Mann T, Brodie BR, Grossman W, McLaurin L. Effusive-constrictive hemodynamic pattern due to neoplastic involvement of the pericardium. *Am J Cardiol* 1978; **41**: 781–6.

7   Sagrista-Sauleda J, Angel J, Permanyer-Miralda G, *et al.* Long-term follow-up of idiopathic chronic pericardial effusion. *N Engl J Med* 1999; **341**(27): 2054–9.

8   Millaire A, de Groote P, De Coulx E, Goullard L, Ducloux G. Treatment of recurrent pericarditis with colchicine. *Eur Heart J* 1994; **15**: 120–4.

9   Vaitkus PT, Herrmann HC, LeWinter MM. Treatment of malignant pericardial effusion. *JAMA* 1994; **272**: 59–64.

10 Maisch B, Ristic AD, Pankuweit S, Neubauer A, Moll R. Neoplastic pericardial effusion. Efficacy and safety of intrapericardial treatment with cisplatin. *Eur Heart J* 2002; **23**: 1625–31.

Acute Palliative Care and Pain Control

43 **Initiating Pain Management**

44 **Neuropathic Cancer Pain**

PROBLEM

43 Initiating Pain Management

Karen Neoh, Michael Bennett

Case history

A 69-year-old man attends the oncology outpatient clinic. He complains of moderate-intensity pain in the right subscapular area, shortness of breath on exertion, and weight loss. He is an ex-miner and an ex-smoker of over 50 pack-years. A staging computed tomography (CT) scan has demonstrated appearances consistent with metastatic lung cancer with bone metastases in his right chest wall. A biopsy confirms small-cell lung cancer and the patient is planned to start carboplatin and etoposide chemotherapy. The patient has been taking regular paracetamol and ibuprofen, but his subscapular chest wall pain persists despite this.

How would you characterize and treat this patient's pain?

How would you advise this patient with regard to pain medication?

How would you manage side effects from pain medication?

Background

How would you characterize and treat this patient's pain?

Pain is defined as an unpleasant sensory and emotional experience associated with actual or potential tissue damage, or described in terms of such damage (IASP 1986).[1] The majority of patients with cancer experience pain, therefore it is important for clinicians to understand the impact pain can have on patients, and endeavour to manage symptoms as quickly and effectively as possible.

On average, cancer patients experience two distinct pains. The first step is a thorough clinical assessment; this should include site, character, radiation, exacerbating or relieving factors, timing and severity (see Table 43.1 for further details).

Table 43.1 'SOCRATES' – a common mnemonic for investigating pain		
S	Site	Where is the pain, or the maximal side of the pain?
O	Onset	When did the pain start, was it sudden or gradual? Is the pain progressive or regressive?
C	Character	What is the pain like? An ache? Stabbing? Sharp?
R	Radiation	Does the pain radiate anywhere?
A	Associations	Any other signs or symptoms associated with the pain such as dyspnoea or nausea
T	Time course	Does the pain follow any pattern?
E	Exacerbating/relieving factors	Does anything change the pain?
S	Severity	How bad is the pain? 1–10, with 10 representing the most severe pain.

A full medication history should be taken, including over the counter or complementary therapies. It is important to establish which medications patients feel have been effective for their symptoms and any side effects experienced, as this may affect compliance.

The World Health Organization (WHO) analgesic ladder provides the basis for initiating and titrating (Figure 43.1). This considers the severity of pain and previous analgesia. For example, strong opioids are indicated if pain is moderate to severe in intensity (with no previous analgesia) *or* if pain has not responded to weaker analgesia.

Simple analgesics include paracetamol and non-steroidal anti-inflammatory drugs (NSAIDs). Weak opioids refer to codeine and tramadol. Strong opioids include morphine, oxycodone, fentanyl and buprenorphine. Adjuvant medications are drugs which were not originally formulated for pain but have been found to be effective in certain situations; these include antidepressants and anticonvulsants.

The patient has been taking regular paracetamol and ibuprofen, but his pain remains moderate in intensity, so he needs stronger analgesia. The first-line weak opioid is usually codeine, which can be administered in combination with paracetamol as co-codamol (30/500 mg, two tablets four times daily).

In patients with good enough performance status (Table 43.2), pain from bone metastases often responds well to radiotherapy. Following radiotherapy there may be a flare-up of pain, and it takes 1–2 weeks before any notable improvement is seen. Patients therefore need to have a minimum prognosis of several weeks to benefit from

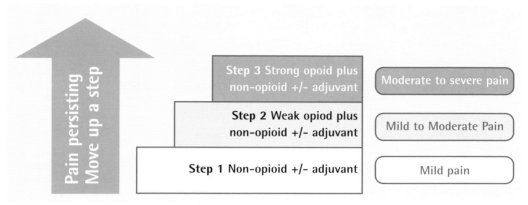

Figure 43.1 World Health Organization (WHO) analgesic ladder.

radiotherapy. A Cochrane review found complete pain relief at one month in 25% of patients and 50% pain relief in 41% of patients following radiotherapy.[2]

Bisphosphonates may be effective in malignant bone pain and can be used in patients with a shorter prognosis.[3] Pain may improve dramatically after treatment with bisphosphonates or radiotherapy, allowing a reduction in the doses of regular analgesia.[4]

The patient calls the lung cancer nurse specialist two weeks after his radiotherapy. He has been taking the co-codamol regularly and has ongoing pain. What do you do next?

How would you advise this patient with regard to pain medication?

In 2012 the National Institute for Health and Care Excellence (NICE) published 'Safe and effective prescribing of strong opioids in palliative care of adults' based on systematic reviews of the best available evidence.[4-6] The recommendations are summarized in the following discussion.

Educational advice and support for patients

It is essential to discuss side effects and common queries associated with opioid medications when commencing treatment. This helps to avoid unnecessary anxiety or worries, e.g. regarding addiction and tolerance. Patients should be told that analgesia will

Table 43.2 The WHO performance status scoring system

Score	Definition
0	Asymptomatic and able to carry on all pre-disease activities
1	Symptomatic but completely ambulatory and independent (restricted in strenuous activities)
2	Symptomatic but less than 50% of time spent in bed during the day (ambulatory and self-caring)
3	Symptomatic and more than 50% of time spent in bed
4	Bedbound and dependent on others completely for all cares
5	Death

be reviewed and that all medication changes will be discussed with their general practitioner (GP) so the patient can seek their GP's help if required.

In addition to verbal advice, written guidance can help to reinforce information. NICE recommend the following should be included:

- when and why strong opioids are used to treat pain
- how effective they are likely to be
- taking strong opioids for background and breakthrough pain, addressing:
  - how, when and how often to take strong opioids
  - how long pain relief should last
- side-effects and signs of toxicity
- safe storage
- follow-up and further prescribing
- information on who to contact out of hours, particularly during initiation of treatment.

Advise patients that it is important to take pain medication regularly to prevent the pain from coming on, rather than waiting until the pain is unbearable. If patients are struggling with oral intake, a change to either liquid form, injection, syringe driver or patches is possible.

Common misconceptions

Many patients may have concerns regarding morphine and other strong opioids. They may feel that once they start taking morphine they are close to the end of life. This is not true, and many patients can take morphine for many years. It can improve quality of life so that people are able to be more active and comfortable. Patients may want to wait until pain is very severe as they may not think that there is anything else once they start taking morphine; hence, patients should be told that doses can be increased, medications can be added, and that there are other forms of pain relief.

The NICE guidance refers to those who require strong opioids (patients in moderate to severe pain) or those whose pain is not controlled by weak opioids. At every stage seek specialist advice if pain is difficult to control or side effects persist. Consider reduced doses or alternative opioids if the patient has moderate to severe hepatic or renal impairment. Adjust the dose to balance pain control and side effects, with frequent review.

Starting strong opioids in those taking oral medication:

1. Titrating the dose

- Offer regular, oral sustained-release or oral immediate-release morphine (depending on patient preference), with rescue doses of oral immediate-release morphine for breakthrough pain.
- Typical daily starting dose of 20-30 mg oral sustained-release morphine given as 10–15 mg twice daily with 5 mg oral immediate-release morphine for breakthrough pain.

2. Maintenance phase

- Offer oral sustained-release morphine as first-line maintenance treatment.
- Offer oral immediate-release morphine for the first-line breakthrough medication.

If oral opioids are not suitable (patients have swallowing problems or if oral absorption is impaired) then:

- consider transdermal patches with the lowest acquisition cost (see Appendix 1 for example calculation)
- consider using subcutaneous opioids with the lowest acquisition cost for patients in whom oral opioids are not suitable and analgesic requirements are unstable.

How would you manage side-effects from pain medication?

1. Inform patients that constipation affects nearly everyone receiving strong opioids and prescribe regular laxative treatment to all patients. Laxatives need to be taken regularly before considering switching to a different strong opioid.

2. Advise patients that nausea may occur when starting strong opioid treatment or when the dose is increased, but that it is likely to be transient. If nausea persists, optimize antiemetic treatment before considering switching to a different opioid.

3. Advise patients that mild drowsiness or impaired concentration may occur when they start strong opioid treatment or when the dose changes, but that these are often transient. Warn patients that impaired concentration may affect their ability to do manual tasks, such as driving.

There is no maximum dose of opioid, but if patients are requiring very high doses reassess the pain and consider alternative causes or non-opioid-sensitive pain. Do not prescribe more than one modified-release opioid at a time. Ensure an immediate-release opioid for episodes of breakthrough pain is prescribed, and patients know that they can take these medications concurrently. The recommended dose of immediate-release morphine for breakthrough pain is the equivalent of up to one-sixth of the total 24-hour morphine dose. For example, a patient talking 60 mg of morphine per 24 hours will usually require 10 mg of morphine for breakthrough pain. Remember to increase this if the long-acting dose is increased.

The patient in this case now needs to progress to step 3 of the analgesic ladder and should be commenced on morphine. This is the strong opioid of choice. Following NICE guidance, a safe and effective staring dose is 15 mg twice daily of sustained-release morphine. This can be titrated according to response at regular follow-up reviews. Meta-analyses show that there is no difference in efficacy or overall side effects between all commonly used strong opioids. However, transdermal preparations (fentanyl and buprenorphine) are associated with moderately less constipation. Individual patients vary in their response to particular strong opioids, so switching to an alternative opioid if side effects persist can sometimes help.

Conclusion

Pain is a commonly experienced symptom in those with cancer. Prompt assessment and initiation of treatment is essential. Imaging may be appropriate to diagnose the cause of pain and therefore to guide the best management of pain. Medications should be increased in a logical stepwise manner, as per the WHO analgesic ladder, with regular reassessment and consideration of the cause of pain. The NICE guideline regarding opioids in palliative care offers advice on starting and titrating strong opioid therapy, but contact with specialist services is advised if pain is uncontrolled or side effects are prominent.

The first-line strong opioid of choice is morphine. When sustained-release-preparations are prescribed an appropriate dose for breakthrough pain should also be prescribed. Side effects should be addressed, and can be avoided with the use of laxatives. If patients cannot take medications by the oral route a topical fentanyl patch can be considered. Alternative routes, such as syringe driver, are available. Patients may have anxieties surrounding opioid use, which should be addressed with verbal and written information. Bone pain can be a particular problem and the use of bisphosphates and radiotherapy is key in such cases.

Further Reading

1　International Association for the Study of Pain. Classification of chronic pain: descriptions of chronic pain syndromes and definitions of pain terms. *Pain Suppl* 1986; 3: S1–S226.

2　McQuay HJ, Collins S, Carroll D, Moore RA. Radiotherapy for the palliation of painful bone metastases. *Cochrane Database Syst Rev* 1999; **3**: CD001793. doi: 10.1002/14651858.CD001793

3　World Health Organization. *Cancer Pain Relief: with a guide to opioid availability.* Geneva: WHO; 1996.

4　Bennett MI, Graham J, Schmidt-Hansen M, Prettyjohns M, Arnold S. Prescribing strong opioids for pain in adult palliative care: summary of NICE guidance. *BMJ* 2012; **344**: e2806.

5　Mannix K, Ahmedzai SH, Anderson H, Bennett M, Lloyd-Williams M, Wilcock A. Using bisphosphonates to control the pain of bone metastases: evidence-based guidelines for palliative care. *Palliative Med* 2000; **14**: 455–61.

6　Caraceni A, Hanks GW, Kaasa S, *et al.* Use of opioid analgesics in the treatment of cancer pain: evidence based recommendations from the EAPC. *Lancet Oncol* 2012; **13**(2): e58–e68.

Appendix 1

Use caution when calculating opioid equivalence for transdermal patches. For example calculating opioid equivalence for transdermal patches:

- a fentanyl 12 µg patch equates to approximately 45 mg oral morphine daily
- a buprenorphine 20 µg patch equates to approximately 30 mg oral morphine daily.

44 Neuropathic Cancer Pain

Adam Hurlow, Michael Bennett

Case history

You are reviewing a 48-year-old woman with recurrent breast cancer following a right-sided mastectomy and chemotherapy she received five years ago. This patient is a candidate for further treatment of ipsilateral supraclavicular nodal and lung involvement. She describes a one-week history of right arm pain and weakness, with constant burning along the medial aspect of the whole limb. She reports a slight reduction in pain with 240 mg of oral codeine phosphate daily. You elicit reduced grip strength and altered sensation in C8–T1 dermatomes.

What is your approach to diagnosis of pain in this patient?

How would you manage this patient's pain?

Background

What is your approach to diagnosis of pain in this patient?

Neuropathic pain should be suspected when a patient describes specific pain qualities in an area of altered sensation consistent with a neuroanatomical distribution.[1] Suggestive descriptors that correlate strongly with altered sensation include 'burning', 'stinging' and 'shooting'.[2]

Neuropathic pain arises as a result of a lesion or disease affecting the central or peripheral somatosensory system.[3] The term encompasses heterogeneous syndromes with diverse aetiologies.[4] The underlying mechanisms are incompletely understood and include: peripheral and central sensitization, neuronal hyperexcitability, maintained sympathetic activity, dysfunctional central inhibition, dorsal horn rewiring, and phenotypic switch.[4]

The prevalence of cancer patients with neuropathic pain ranges between 19% and 39%, with 19%–24% of all pains having a neuropathic mechanism.[5] Cancer pain typically arises from mixed nociceptive and neuropathic mechanisms, with pain considered more or less neuropathic.[6,7] Failure to identify a neuropathic component may contribute to the under-treatment of pain.[5]

Approximately two-thirds of neuropathic cancer pain arises from the cancer itself, through direct invasion or paraneoplastic neuropathy, with 20% arising from anticancer treatment. Up to 10% reflects comorbidity.[5] In the absence of previous radiotherapy, brachial plexopathy secondary to metastatic involvement is likely in this case.

Patients may describe or exhibit the following:[1,8]

- pain occurring without a precipitating trigger (spontaneous pain), like shooting electrical attacks (paroxysmal pain)
- numbness or reduced sensation to painful (hypoalgesia) and non-painful stimuli (hypoaesthesia)
- unusual and unpleasant sensations, such as tingling or pins and needles (dysaesthesia/paraesthesia)
- pain responses to usually non-painful stimuli (allodynia)
- exaggerated response to usually painful stimuli (hyperalgesia)
- abnormal thermal sensation.

Clinical examination focuses on identifying abnormal sensation in the area of pain. Allodynia is demonstrated by eliciting pain through gentle brushing (normally non-painful). Response to pin-prick testing may be reduced (numbness) or exaggerated (hyperalgesia). Temporal summation, in which there is increasing pain sensation with repetitive application of identical stimuli, is demonstrated by repeated pin-pricks with intervals of under 3 seconds for 30 seconds.[1,8]

Although assessment tools exist there are no universally accepted and validated diagnostic criteria for neuropathic cancer pain.[1,5,8] Diagnosis is usually clinical and can be graded with regard to the criteria in Table 44.1. Imaging, neurophysiology and blood tests are indicated where there is diagnostic uncertainty and findings would alter management.[1] In the case presented here, clinical findings are consistent with brachial plexopathy, and metastatic infiltration of the plexus is plausible given the distribution of recurrence.

Table 44.1: Criteria to be evaluated for the diagnosis of neuropathic pain. (Adapted from ref. 3.)

	Grading of certainty for the presence of neuropathic pain:		
1 Pain with a neuroanatomically plausible distribution	Possible neuropathic pain: 1 and 2, without 3 or 4		
2 A history suggestive of a relevant lesion or disease affecting the peripheral or central somatosensory system		Probable neuropathic pain: 1 and 2, plus either 3 or 4	
3 Demonstration of altered sensation in the distribution of pain by at least one bedside test, e.g. allodynia, hyperalgesia, numbness			Definite neuropathic pain: all criteria fulfilled (1 to 4)
4 Demonstration of the relevant lesion or disease by at least one confirmatory test, e.g. tumour plexus invasion on MRI or CT			

CT, computed tomography; MRI, magnetic resonance imaging.

How would you manage this patient's pain?

Neuropathic cancer pain can be controlled in the majority of patients (86%–95%) following the multimodal approach set out in the World Health Organization (WHO) analgesic ladder.[9,10] This advises stepwise titration of opioids, with the addition of adjuvants (agents exerting analgesic effects, although this is not their primary indication), non-opioid analgesics and non-pharmacological measures at any stage.

Although opioids can be an effective monotherapy for neuropathic cancer pain – up to 47% of patients may not require adjuvants – higher doses may be necessary.[4,9] Following WHO guidelines, between 53% and 70% of patients required an adjuvant, with 12% managed using adjuvants only.[9,10] The addition of an antidepressant or anticonvulsant to opioid therapy improves cancer pain control, but can cause significantly more adverse effects unless both drugs are at doses lower than used in monotherapy.[11] The reduction in pain intensity may be no greater than one point on a 0–10 scale, with any benefit seen within four to eight days.[11] A recent Cochrane review found multiple good-quality studies demonstrating superior efficacy of two-drug combinations in cancer and non-cancer neuropathic pain. There was insufficient evidence to recommend particular combinations.[12]

Adjuvants with the most robust evidence base in non-cancer neuropathic pain are the tricyclic antidepressants (TCAs: amitriptyline, nortriptyline) and anticonvulsants (pregabalin and gabapentin).[1,13,14] These drugs work through different pharmacological mechanisms and may act synergistically in combination.[11,12] However, combining drugs with similar mechanisms of action (e.g. pregabalin and gabapentin, or two TCAs) should be avoided.

The use of corticosteroids for neuropathic pain from malignant nerve compression is established practice, especially when there is associated weakness.[15] There is some evidence, albeit limited, for corticosteroids in neuropathic cancer pain, particularly from malignant spinal cord compression.[16] Their efficacy is time-limited and side effects complicate prolonged use.[16] Corticosteroid use allows time for definitive treatment or titration of other agents. Topical agents warrant consideration as they lack systematic adverse effects. Lidocaine 5% topical patches may have a role for peripheral, well circumscribed, cutaneous neuropathic pain associated with allodynia.[17]

A variety of other agents have been used, including NMDA receptor antagonists, cannabinoids and intravenous local anaesthetics. They are not considered first- or second-line agents for a variety of reasons, including a lack of robust evidence, use in specific circumstances, problematic toxicities, or complex titration.[4] The number needed to treat (NNT) and number needed to harm (NNH) for recommended agents is provided in Table 44.2. The figures are derived from non-cancer pain studies, and, given the frailty of cancer patients, it is likely that NNH will be lower and NNT higher in this population.[11]

In the case reported above there has been a limited response to codeine phosphate, suggesting the patient's pain is at least partially opioid sensitive. Conversion to regular modified-release oral morphine, with immediate-release morphine for breakthrough pain, is an appropriate next step. Dexamethasone should be started simultaneously at 8 mg. Given its 36–54 hour duration of action, a single morning dose of dexamethasone is advised to minimize sleep disruption.[19] Should pain persist despite opioid titration, addition of either a low-dose TCA (amitriptyline 10 mg at night) or anticonvulsant

Table 44.2 Numbers needed to treat (NNT) and harm (NNH) for recommended medication derived from studies in non-cancer neuropathic pain [18]

Medication	NNT for 50% pain relief (95% CI)	NNH for study withdrawal (95% CI)
TCAs	2.1 (1.8–2.6) to 3.1(2.2–5.5)*	14.7 (10.2–25.2)
Gabapentin	3.8 (3.1–5.1) to 5.1 (4.1–6.8)†	26.1 (14.1–170)
Pregabalin	3.7 (3.2–4.4)	7.4 (6.0–9.5)
Morphine	2.5 (1.9–3.4)	17.1(10–66)¶
Oxycodone	2.6 (1.9–4.1)	

* NNT varies with neuropathic pain type treated.
† NNT varies with dose schedule, lower NNT with higher doses.
¶ NNH for morphine and oxycodone combined.

(pregabalin 25 mg twice daily, or gabapentin 100–300 mg thrice daily) is appropriate. The opioid dose should be reviewed and may need adjustment. The benefit of any addition should be assessed within a week, and dose titration or a switch to an alternative adjuvant may be considered. Consultation with pain specialists is advised when prescribing unfamiliar medication, when pain is severe or refractory to the approach described or adverse effects limit tolerability.

A proportion of neuropathic cancer pain is refractory to pharmacotherapy.[4] Where possible the causative lesion should be treated. In this case radiotherapy, chemotherapy or endocrine therapy may be indicated.[20] Invasive anaesthetic interventions, a brachial plexus block, for example, may have a role.[21] The psycho social context and multidimensional determinants of pain should be managed through physiotherapy, occupational therapy, psychological and existential spiritual input.[4]

Conclusion

Management of neuropathic cancer pain is multimodal and likely to require polypharmacy. The role of opioids and adjuvants, including which to use as first-line therapy, in what combination and at what dose, remains contentious. Pharmacotherapy should be tailored to the individual taking into account patient preferences, sensitivities, concurrent medication and comorbidities. For instance, TCAs should be avoided in a patient with a history of cardiac dysrhythmias. Evidence supports the WHO analgesic ladder for initial management of neuropathic pain. It is prudent to introduce one agent at a time, minimizing polypharmacy, and facilitating attribution of benefit or adverse effect to a particular medication. When used in combination agents should be started at low doses, the efficacy of combinations should be reviewed within a week, and medication should be reduced to the minimum effective dose.

Further reading

1 Freynhagen R, Bennett MI. Diagnosis and management of neuropathic pain. *BMJ* 2009; **339**: 391–5.

2 Holtan A, Kongsgaard UE. The use of pain descriptors in cancer patients. *J Pain Symptom Manage* 2009; **38**: 208–15.

3   Treede DR, Jensen ST, Campbell NJ, *et al.* Neuropathic pain: redefinition and a grading system for clinical and research purposes. *Neurology* 2008; **7**: 1630–5.

4   Vadalouca A, Raptis E, Moka E, *et al.* Pharmacological treatment of neuropathic cancer pain: a comprehensive view of the current literature. *Pain Pract* 2011; **12**: 219–51.

5   Bennett MI, Rayment C, Hjermstad M, *et al.* Prevalence and aetiology of neuropathic pain in cancer patients: a systematic review. *Pain* 2012; **153**: 359–65.

6   Mercadente S, Gebbia V, David F, *et al.* Tools for identifying cancer pain of predominantly neuropathic origin and opioid responsiveness in cancer patients. *J Pain* 2009; **6**: 594–600.

7   Bennett MI, Smith HB, Torrance N, *et al.* Can pain be more or less neuropathic: comparison of symptom assessment tools with ratings of certainty by clinicians. *Pain* 2006; **122**: 289–94.

8   Baron R, Binder A, Wasner G. Neuropathic pain: diagnosis, pathophysiological mechanisms, and treatment. *Lancet Neurol* 2010; **9**: 807–19.

9   Grond S, Radbruch L, Meuser T, *et al.* Assessment and treatment of neuropathic cancer pain following WHO guidelines. *Pain* 1999; **79**: 15–20.

10   Mishra S, Bhatnagar S, Gupta D, *et al.* Management of neuropathic cancer pain following WHO analgesic ladder: A prospective study. *Am J Hosp Palliat Care* 2009; **25**: 447–51.

11   Bennett MI. Effectiveness of antiepileptic or antidepressant drugs when added to opioids for cancer pain: systematic review. *Palliat Med* 2010; **25**: 553–9.

12   Chaparro LE, Wiffen PJ, Moore RA, Gilron I. Combination pharmacotherapy for the treatment of neuropathic pain in adults. *Cochrane Database Syst Rev* 2012; **7**: CD008943.

13   EFNS guidelines on the pharmacological treatment of neuropathic pain: 2010 revision. *Eur J Neurol* 2010; **17**: 1113–23.

14   National Institute for Health and Clinical Excellence [Internet]. Neuropathic pain: the pharmacological management of neuropathic pain in adults in non-specialist settings (CG96). London: National Institute for Health and Care Excellence. c.2013. [Issued Mar 2010]. Available from: www.nice.org.uk/cg96

15   Lussier D, Huskey AG, Portenoy RK. Adjuvant analgesics in cancer pain management. *Oncologist* 2004; **9**: 571–91.

16   Watanbe S, Bruera E. Corticosteroids as adjuvant analgesics. *J Pain Symptom Manage* 199; **9**: 442–5.

17   Fleming JA, O'Connor BD. Use of lidocaine plasters for neuropathic pain in a comprehensive cancer centre. *Pain Res Manag* 2009; **14**: 381–8.

18   Finnerup NB, Otto M, Jensen TS, *et al.* An evidence-based algorithm for the treatment of neuropathic pain. *MedGenMed* 2007; **9**(2): 36.

19   Twycross R, Wilcock A, editors-in-chief. *Palliative Care Formulary.* 4th ed. Nottingham: Palliativedrugs.com Ltd; 2011: pp.483–93.

20   Kamenova B, Braverman AS, Schwartz M, *et al.* Effective treatment of the brachial plexus syndrome in breast cancer patients by early detection and control of loco-regional metastases with radiation or systemic therapy. *Int J Clin Oncol* 2009; **14**: 219–24.

21   Hicks F, Simpson KH. *Nerve blocks in palliative care.* Oxford University Press; 2004: pp.57–63.

Patients in Clinical Trials

PROBLEM

45 Management of Acute Toxicity of Patients in Clinical Trials

Adel Jebar, Chris Twelves, Debbie Beirne

Case History

The concerned wife of a 54-year-old man calls the acute oncology unit. She tells you that her husband has brain cancer, and has recently started an experimental tablet at your hospital as part of a small clinical trial that will include only a few patients. She thinks he has had a fit lasting approximately three minutes, but appears to be recovering now. His last fit was one year ago, several months prior to commencing the trial.

The patient is taking part in a small trial, possibly phase I. It is difficult to determine from the information presented whether the drug is previously untested in patients (a first-in-humans study), or whether it has been previously tested and is now being given for a new indication. If the latter is true, more information regarding the expected side effects may already be available.

What is a clinical trial and who may participate?

Where should patients involved in trials be admitted acutely?

How should patients in trials be managed?

Background

Clinical research is central to oncology, and in the UK as many as 20% of patients may be enrolled into clinical studies. Such patients may experience acute episodes, possibly due to the study treatments. In early clinical trials these may be new or unexpected events.

Patients in trials who present acutely may therefore be especially challenging for the acute oncology team (AOT).

What is a clinical trial and who may participate?

Clinical trials are generally considered to be biomedical or health-related research studies in human beings that follow a predefined protocol. In oncology, the majority of these clinical trials are interventional, with patients assigned to a treatment or other intervention. Observational studies are those in which individuals are observed without intervention in order to measure predefined outcomes.[1]

All clinical trials have guidelines, including inclusion and exclusion criteria that define who can participate. These criteria not only help to keep the participants safe, but they also help to identify appropriate participants to ensure that researchers will be able to answer the questions they plan to study.[2] Examples of criteria include the type and stage of the cancer, molecular characteristics of their tumour (including genetic mutations), previous treatment history, and other medical conditions.

Clinical trials are traditionally conducted in four phases, each of which has a different purpose and help to answer different questions.[3,4] Table 45.1 lists the approximate number of participants and primary and secondary measures (endpoints) for each phase of a clinical trial.

Table 45.1 The four phases of clinical trials in oncology

Phase	Typical number and type of participants	Primary end points	Secondary end points
I	10–60; may have a range of different advanced cancers or be more limited	1) Determine maximum tolerated dose of a new agent and establish the dose/schedule to be taken forward in later trials 2) Evaluate safety and side-effect profile	1) Pharmacokinetics (measurements of drug levels in blood or other tissues) 2) Pharmacodynamics (molecular markers of drug activity in tumour or surrogate tissues) 3) Early indications of anti-tumour activity
II	50–150; usually patients with specific type(s) of cancer	1) Establish evidence of anti-tumour activity to inform subsequent Phase III trials	1) Confirm tolerability and side effects 2) Establish potential of biomarkers to predict treatment effects
III	300–3000; patients with specific types of cancer randomized to receive the new treatment or standard treatment	1) Determine superiority/ equivalence in terms of efficacy compared to standard treatments 2) Inform progress towards application for licensing	1) Compare side effects 2) Compare quality of life with the new treatment compared to standard treatment 3) Examine cost-effectiveness of the new and standard treatments
IV	Ongoing	1) Post-marketing studies to determine the drug's risks, benefits and optimal use	

Where should patients involved in trials be admitted acutely?

In 2011, nearly a quarter of patients with cancer took part in a clinical trial, some of these trials involve the use of investigational agents, not previously licensed.[5] When taking a call from a relative or a patient, always be aware of this and ask the name of the trial, the name of the study agent, and when the patient last took it. Do they have any written information about the trial to hand?

Patients on trials can sometimes be given advice over the telephone, but as the patient in this case may well be taking an unlicensed drug with unpredictable side effects, there should be a low threshold for reviewing him in hospital. The next consideration is where to admit the patient. If his nearest hospital is the one where the trial is being run, that is where he should be admitted. However, because not all trials are available at every hospital, patients may live far away from where the trial is being run; depending on the urgency of the situation, it may be wise to arrange urgent review at hospital local to the patient, ideally in an oncology unit. It is vital to ensure good communication between the admitting hospital and the centre where the trial is being coordinated.[6] Patients enrolled on a clinical trial should be provided with a 24-hour telephone contact for the research team; the attending clinician can use that number to contact the research team.[7] If it is recommended that the patient be admitted to another hospital, then the attending clinician should speak to the clinical team under whom the patient is admitted; likewise, the admitting hospital should contact the trial team to inform them of the patient's admission. In both circumstances it is important the admitting hospital seek advice over the patient's management from the study centre. The trial team also have an obligation to inform the central trial organizers within 24 hours of hearing that a patient has been admitted.[8]

How should patients in trials be managed?

Wherever possible, you should seek appropriate information and advice prior to instigating a treatment plan. The patient's acute problems may be side effects of the trial drug and require specific management. Also, treatment you would ordinarily use to treat a particular problem may interact with trial drugs. Protocol-related guidance should be sought and adhered to. Where following the protocol might put the patient at risk, advice should be obtained from the local principal investigator or named medical contact of the sponsor coordinating the study.

Clinical trial protocols describe the study agent, expected toxicities, symptom management algorithms and any other guidance arising from preclinical data. For example, do not assume that a patient with diarrhoea is suffering from chemotherapy-related expected toxicity: it may be an autoimmune effect of an immune modulator and could lead to serious inflammatory bowel complications including perforation. This requires specific management, which will be detailed in the protocol. The Investigator Brochure (IB) for each investigational agent contains a more detailed summary of all adverse events and is regularly updated.

In the current era of targeted therapies, extra care must be taken to avoid drug–drug interactions. Trial protocols have a section describing those medications that are permitted, those to be used with caution, and prohibited medications. These represent, for example, drugs that may slow down the elimination of an investigational agent, thus increasing the risk of toxicity. It may be necessary to administer medication that is normally precluded by the protocol, but, again, such decisions should be taken by senior colleagues in consultation with the investigator and/or study sponsors. After such advice, it may also be appropriate to stop the investigational agent while managing the acute event.

Randomized trials may involve patients being allocated (or randomized) to an investigational agent, standard therapy or placebo. Sometimes, neither the patient, nor the investigators know which the patient is taking (a process known as 'blinding'). Patients taking part in such trials may pose particular challenges to the medical team if they present acutely. Where possible, they should be managed in a way that takes into account the possibility of their having received any of the drugs available on the trial.[6] If, however, the patient's safety is a concern, the identity of the study drug can be revealed, usually by consulting the pharmacy department in the hospital who will keep appropriate records (a process known as 'unblinding').

It is particularly important to ensure that documentation in the medical notes is clear and thorough, as this will be used to guide accurate reporting of the adverse event by the study team. Any admission to hospital must be reported to the study sponsor as a 'serious adverse event' within 24 hours of being made aware of it.[8] Informing the research team in a timely manner is essential to fulfill the requirement for good clinical practice (GCP). The medical notes may also be audited by the regulatory bodies as an investigational agent progresses towards licensing.

Conclusions

1. Many patients take part in clinical trials of investigational agents, so always consider the possibility when assessing an acute admission.
2. The trial protocol must be available at the hospital where the trial is being conducted, and contains important information about potential toxicities, how they should be managed, and potential drug interactions.
3. It is important to contact, consult and work with the clinical team conducting the study, who should be contacted in a timely manner.
4. The patient's safety is the overriding concern. Accurate note keeping is vital, and ready access to the protocol and IB are essential aspects of safe practice.
5. Where adverse events occur, it is essential to inform the trial investigators. This is not only for the further management of your patient, but also to ensure that the investigators gain a picture of possible toxicities to inform their safe management of the trial.

Further Reading

1 ClinicalTrials.gov. *Learn About Clinical Studies* [Internet]. Bethesda: National Library of Medicine; Aug 2012. Available at: http://clinicaltrials.gov/ct2/about-studies/learn

2 CancerHelp UK. *Trials and Research* [Internet]. London: Cancer Research UK; Sep 2012. Available at: www.cancerresearchuk.org [Homepage]

3 ClinicalTrials.gov. *Protocol Data Element Definitions (DRAFT)* [Internet]. Bethesda: National Library of Medicine; Jan 2013. Available at: http://prsinfo.clinicaltrials.gov/definitions.html#StudyPhase

4   Eisenhauer EA, Twelves C, Buyse M. *Phase 1 Cancer Clinical Trials: A Practical Guide.* Oxford
     University Press; 26 July 2006. 343p.

5   National Institute for Health Research Cancer Research Network (NCRN) [Homepage].
     Leeds: National Cancer Research Network; c.2011. Available at: www.ncrn.org.uk

6   Mort D, Lansdown M, Smith N, Protopapa K, Mason M. 2008. *For better, for worse? A review
     of the care of patients who died within 30 days of receiving systemic anti-cancer therapy.* London:
     National Confidential Enquiry into Patient Outcome and Death (NCEPOD); Nov 2008. 150p.

7   National Chemotherapy Advisory Group. *Chemotherapy Services in England: Ensuring quality
     and safety.* London: Department of Health; 21 Aug 2009. 70p. Available at: www.dh.gov.uk
     [Homepage]

8   ICH Steering Committee. *ICH Harmonised Tripartite Guideline. Guideline for Good
     Clinical Practice E6(R1). Step 4 Version.* Geneva: International Conference on
     Harmonisation of Technical Requirements for Registration of Pharmaceuticals for Human
     Use; 10 Jun 1996. 59p.

46 Recording and Reporting Adverse Events in the Context of Clinical Trials

Adel Jebar, Chris Twelves, Debbie Beirne

Case History

A 69-year-old woman with metastatic breast cancer is admitted to hospital overnight with a history of haematemesis; she has no previous history of gastrointestinal (GI) problems. The patient says she is taking part in a trial comparing chemotherapy against an investigational oral drug (or placebo), and last took the study drug that morning. On admission, she is hypotensive and requires resuscitation with blood and intravenous fluids; she undergoes an upper GI endoscopy that shows a bleeding duodenal ulcer. The following morning the patient has stabilized, and the research nurse asks you to complete an assessment of this event as part of your responsibility as a named sub-investigator on the trial.

How would you assess and record this patient's acute event?

How would you report adverse events in a case like this?

Background

Clinical trials are conducted by local teams of doctors, nurses and support staff, led by the 'Principal Investigator' (PI). A sub-investigator is a member of the clinical trial team (usually a doctor or a research nurse) who is designated to perform critical trial-related procedures and/or to make important trial-related decisions.[1] Anyone involved in the conduct of clinical trials must be trained in the principles of clinical trial practice. These principles have been agreed internationally, and are bound by both international and UK law.

The International Conference on Harmonisation of Good Clinical Practice (ICH-GCP) guideline is an international ethical and scientific quality standard for designing, conducting, recording and reporting trials that involve the participation of human subjects.[2] The objective of the ICH-GCP guideline is to provide a unified international standard to facilitate the mutual acceptance of clinical data by the various regulatory authorities. Compliance with GCP provides assurance that the rights, safety and well-being of trial subjects are protected, and that the results of the clinical trials are credible. Prospective PIs and sub-investigators must complete training in ICH-GCP and may be required to pass an examination prior to involvement in clinical trials.

Fundamental to the conduct of clinical trials is the protection of human rights and the dignity of human beings, as reflected in the 1996 version of the Declaration of Helsinki.[3] In the UK, the Department of Health has published detailed documents for the governance of clinical research undertaken in the NHS. These are the 'Research Governance Framework for Health and Social Care' and 'The Medicines for Human Use (Clinical Trials) Regulations 2004'.[4,5]

Trial participants are protected through risk assessment by various competent authorities prior to the commencement of a clinical trial. These include the judgement of the Main Research Ethics Committee (MREC),[6] and if the trial involves a medicine or a medical device, permission from the Medicines and Healthcare Products Regulatory Agency (MHRA) would also be required.[7]

How would you assess and record this patient's acute event?

One of the most important aims of all clinical trials that involve medicines is to collect data on the investigational drug's side effects. Therefore, the assessment and documentation of toxicity experienced by patients such as the one in the above scenario forms an important part of the duties of a sub-investigator. When assisting the study nurse/research staff to complete the initial report of this patient's event, it is important to record the clinical observations clearly and fully. This includes documenting when symptoms developed (and then resolved), recording the investigations and interventions undertaken, as well as recording the outcomes.

An adverse event (AE) is defined as 'any untoward medical occurrence in a patient or clinical investigation subject administered a pharmaceutical product and that does not necessarily have a causal relationship to this treatment'.[8] An adverse reaction (AR) implies a causal relationship to the study drug. All AEs and ARs have to be recorded in the patient's medical records and will then be transcribed onto a case record form (CRF). The CRF is a paper or electronic record of all events related to the patient while participating in a trial. A serious adverse event/reaction (SAE/R) is an AE or AR that 'at any dose results in death, is life-threatening, requires hospitalization or prolongation of existing hospitalization'.[8] Further trial-specific definitions will be listed in the protocol.

This patient's episode of haematemesis is clearly an SAE/SAR in that it was both life-threatening and required hospitalization; hypotension and anaemia may also be recorded in the initial report as secondary adverse events. Hospitalization in the context of an SAE/SAR usually implies formal admission for inpatient care. If a patient attends hospital for assessment, that in itself would not constitute the episode being an SAE; the investigator would, however, need to exercise their judgement in deciding whether to record it as an SAE, taking into account the seriousness of the situation, and any treatment instituted.

Next you need to assess the severity of the event; this is quite distinct from whether the AE was 'serious' as described above. In trials, the severity of an AE is graded using the Common Terminology Criteria for Adverse Events (CTCAE);[9] again, a listing of the CTCAE grades will be part of the protocol, often as an appendix. Most CTCAE grades have a 5-point scale: e.g. 'Haemorrhage GI' is graded from 1 (mild, intervention [other than iron supplements] not indicated) to 5 (death). This patient's AE would be graded 3 (transfusion, interventional radiography, endoscopic, or operative intervention indicated, i.e. haemostasis of bleeding site).

You also need to make a judgement as to whether the study drug may have been responsible for this SAE.[8] Again, refer to the study protocol for guidance, but the initial question may be whether or not there is a 'reasonable possibility' that the event was related to the study drug, to which you would answer 'yes' in this case and record the event as a SAR. More detailed attribution may take the form of a series of options from 'unrelated' to 'definitely related'. For this patient, you would judge the event as 'probably related' to the study drug, especially as she had no prior history of GI disease.

Finally, you should check whether this particular toxicity is consistent in nature and severity with information in the current Clinical Investigator Brochure (IB). If it is not, the event should be considered a suspected unexpected serious adverse reaction (SUSAR).[8] For example, should the IB not mention that the study drug can cause GI bleeding, you would need to consider recording this patient's event as a SUSAR. Table 46.1 summarizes the definitions of the various untoward medical occurrences. Further study-specific guidance will be present in the trial protocol.

Table 46.1 Definitions used for reporting adverse events involving drugs in clinical trials			
Untoward medical occurrence	Causality to study drug	Seriousness	Event previously reported in the IB?
AE – Adverse event	Unlikely to be related	Non-life-threatening and does not require hospitalization	Yes
AR – Adverse reaction	May have been caused by the study drug	Non-life-threatening and does not require hospitalization	Yes
SAE – Serious adverse event	Unlikely to be related	Results in death, is life-threatening or requires hospitalization	Yes
SAR – Serious adverse reaction	May have been caused by the study drug	Results in death, is life-threatening or requires hospitalization	Yes
SUSAR – Suspected unexpected serious adverse reaction	May have been caused by the study drug	Results in death, is life-threatening or requires hospitalization	No

As this patient is taking part in a blinded trial, accurately documenting their acute event may require that we know exactly which drug they are taking. Given that this patient's toxicity was serious, there are important consequences for other patients taking part in the same trial, who may be exposed to the ongoing risk of similar harm without their knowledge or that of their treating medical team. It may therefore be prudent to consider unblinding this patient's treatment in consultation with the PI and trial sponsor.

After the initial SAE form has been completed, follow-up forms may be submitted as more information becomes available.[8]

How would you report adverse events in a case like this?

Adverse events and adverse reactions should be recorded as described above, but the sponsor does not need to be notified of these and they do not need to be sent routinely to the MREC or MHRA. Serious adverse events must be reported to the sponsor within 24 hours of the investigator becoming aware of them, so there is a need to provide as much information as possible within this time frame.[8] If this patient's haematemesis is prolonged, further follow-up reporting is required until such time as the toxicity is resolved or no further change/improvement is expected.

The PI should be made aware of all SAEs, SARs and SUSARs as soon as possible.[8] It is the responsibility of the PI to report these immediately to the sponsor. The sponsor is responsible for periodically sending a collated list of SAEs and SARs to the MHRA and MREC. For SUSARs, these are subject to expedited reporting. For fatal or life-threatening events this is within seven days of hearing of the event. For non-fatal, non-life-threatening events these are required to be reported within 15 days of the event.

Conclusions

1 The conduct of clinical trials is governed by national and international laws and regulations. You should be familiar with these regulations prior to becoming involved in clinical trials.

2 You should assess a patient's acute event according to its seriousness, causality and expectedness.

3 The principal investigator must report serious events to the sponsor, who in turn is responsible for reporting these to the competent authorities.

Further Reading

1 ICH Steering Committee. *ICH Harmonised Tripartite Guideline. Guideline for Good Clinical Practice E6(R1). Step 4 Version.* Geneva: International Conference on Harmonisation of Technical Requirements for Registration of Pharmaceuticals for Human Use; 10 Jun 1996. 59p.

2 The International Conference on Harmonisation of Technical Requirements for Registration of Pharmaceuticals for Human Use (ICH) [Homepage]. Geneva: ICH; c.2013. Available at www.ich.org

3 WMA Declaration of Helsinki – Ethical Principles for Medical Research Involving Human Subjects. Ferney-Voltaire, France: World Medical Association; Oct 2008. Available at: www.wma.net [Homepage]

4 Department of Health. *Research governance framework for health and social care.* 2nd ed. London: Department of Health; Apr 2005. Available from: www.dh.gov.uk

5 The Medicines for Human Use (Clinical Trials) Regulations 2004, SI 2004/1031. Available from: www.legislation.gov.uk

6 National Research Ethics Service [Homepage]. London: Health Research Authority; c.2013. Available from: www.nres.nhs.uk

7 Medicines and Healthcare products Regulatory Agency [Homepage]. Crown copyright; c.2013. Available from: www.mhra.gov.uk

8 Detailed guidance on the collection, verification and presentation of adverse reaction reports arising from clinical trials on medicinal products for human use ('CT-3'). [2011] *OJ* C172/01. Available from: http://ec.europa.eu

9 National Institutes of Health, National Cancer Institute. *Common Terminology Criteria for Adverse Events, version 4.03.* NIH publication no.09-5410 [revised Jun 2010]. Bethesda: National Institutes of Health; 14 Jun 2010. Available from: http://ctep.cancer.gov

47 Informed Consent in Clinical Trials: A Dynamic Process

Adel Jebar, Chris Twelves, Debbie Beirne

Case History

During an outpatient clinic, the next patient is a 35-year-old woman with metastatic sarcoma who has been taking part in a phase II clinical trial of a new intravenous investigational agent. Following her first dose, she suffered from neutropenic sepsis and severe diarrhoea, and required support on the high dependency unit. During the consultation, with a clinician who is a named sub-investigator in the trial, the patient informs the clinician that she would like to continue taking part in the trial.

The definition of informed consent according to The Medicines for Human Use (Clinical Trials) Regulations 2004 is that 'a person gives informed consent to take part in a clinical trial only if his/her decision is given freely after that person is informed of the nature, significance, implications and risks of the trial'.[1]

When and how should informed consent be taken for patients in clinical trials?

Does this patient's toxicity affect the validity of consent for other patients in the same trial?

Background

When and how should informed consent be taken for patients in clinical trials?

This patient will have given and recorded her consent to take part in the trial prior to any study-specific intervention. That would usually suffice. However, given that she has clearly suffered from a serious event, it is important to undertake further detailed discussions to ensure that if she does wish to remain in the trial, she does so with her fully informed consent.

The process of valid informed consent to research participation is a continuous one. Following an adverse event such as this, it is important that the patient understands clearly what has occurred and, where it is possible to establish, why it occurred. This will inform discussion about the most appropriate management thereafter, including possible dose interruption, reduction or withdrawal from the study. The patient should be aware that they are free to withdraw from the study at any time without giving an explanation.[2]

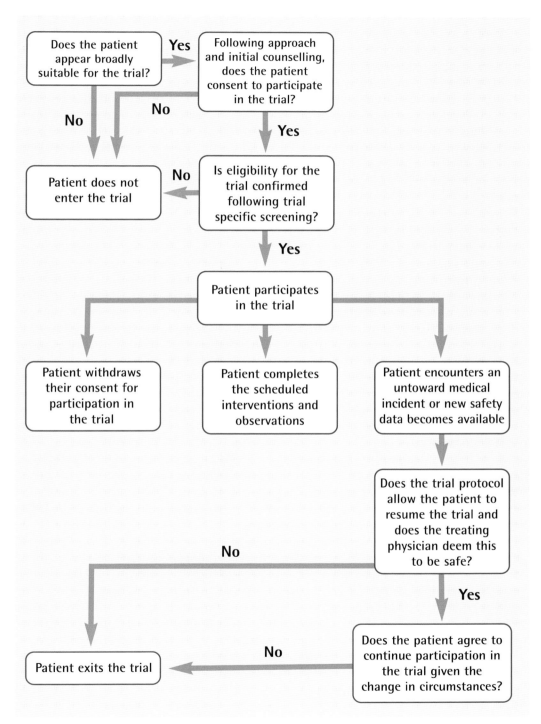

Figure 47.1 Process of obtaining informed consent both at the beginning of the trial and at subsequent points of contact with the investigators.

Whether the patient resumes treatment within the study following resolution or acceptable improvement of the adverse event will depend on several factors, including those mandated in the trial protocol. Important considerations are the Common Terminology Criteria for Adverse Events (CTCAE) grade of the event, level of intervention required and length of time to resolution; but also included is the medical judgement of the responsible physician. Likewise, the protocol will usually define changes to the dose or schedule of study drug if the patient remains on the trial. Again, the investigator has the responsibility to ensure that, if implemented, such changes in the study drug are in the patient's best interest. The patient's own wishes are also important.

Does this patient's toxicity affect the validity of consent for other patients in the same trial?

Following this episode, as a sub-investigator you may be involved in informed consent discussions with prospective patients, or those already enrolled in the study. Informing patients of known adverse events that occur within a study is an integral part of the informed consent process. The patient information sheet (PIS) that all patients receive, and should read and understand before signing the consent form, will list expected possible toxicities. Nevertheless, the investigator has an obligation to provide additional information as it becomes available once the trial is under way. Indeed, it is not uncommon for patients to enquire about toxicity seen to date. Where there has been severe, unexpected toxicity the PIS may need to be amended to take this into account. Other patients that are already established in the same trial should be informed of the change, and asked to reconfirm their informed consent. In other situations where additional information is given to the patient, the investigator should record in the case notes what was said, by whom and when. Figure 47.1 summarizes the informed consent process for patients in trials.

Conclusions

1. The process of informed consent for trial patients is a continuous one. When a patient's circumstances change, or when new pertinent information comes to light, the patient's informed consent should be confirmed.
2. New information may have important implications on the validity of informed consent for other patients in the same trial.

Further Reading

1   The Medicines for Human Use (Clinical Trials) Regulations 2004, SI 2004/1031. Available from: www.legislation.gov.uk

2   General Medical Council [Internet]. *Good practice in research: Consent to research*. London: General Medical Council; c.2013. Available from: www.gmc-uk.org/guidance

Index